THE BEST
BABY
NAMES
for BOYS

EMILY LARSON

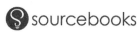

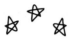

Published by Sourcebooks.
P.O. Box 4410, Naperville, Illinois 60567-4410
(630) 961-3900
sourcebooks.com

Library of Congress Cataloging-in-Publication Data

Names: Larson, Emily, author.
Title: The best baby names for boys : the ultimate resource for finding the
    perfect boy / Emily Larson.
Description: Naperville : Sourcebooks, IL [2019]
Identifiers: LCCN 2019008402 | (trade pbk. : alk. paper)
Subjects: LCSH: Names, Personal--Dictionaries. | Masculine
    names--Dictionaries.
Classification: LCC CS2377 .L388 2019 | DDC 929.403--dc23 LC record available at https://lccn.loc
.gov/2019008402

Printed and bound in the United States of America.
SB 10 9 8 7 6 5 4 3 2 1

Contents

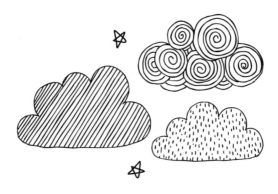

Introduction

Congratulations, you're having a little boy! And now that you've discovered the gender (or even if you haven't yet and are just hoping!) it's time to buckle down and sift through the countless options available to you until you find the perfect name! But where do you even begin? Boys' names can be tricky, and the options (and opinions) are endless. As if preparing for the arrival of a baby isn't stressful enough, you are now under the added pressure of giving your child a name that he will have to live with for the rest of his life. Add to that the never-ending suggestions from well-meaning family and friends—and possibly a few arguments with your partner—and baby naming can become quite the daunting task! But it doesn't have to be. Believe it or not, you can actually have fun with the baby-naming process, and this book is here to help. Why browse through a massive compendium of baby names (half of which won't even apply to your child!) when you can breeze through *The Best Baby*

Names for Boys and discover the perfect option for your family? And even if you've gone through all of the lists and still haven't found the perfect fit, advice and journaling prompts appear throughout to help guide you to discovering the perfect little boy name for *your* family.

Yes, names influence first impressions. Yes, names sometimes spawn not-so-flattering nicknames that can follow a person all the way through retirement. Yes, names affect children's self-esteem. Yes, names are often obligatory ties to family. And yes, there are thousands to choose from. But what you must keep in mind is that this decision is yours. If you choose a name you take great pride in, your child will be proud of his name as well.

Of course, choosing a name requires some forethought—and therefore work—on your part. Even if you've had a name picked out since you were six years old, it is still a good idea to look around. Your child might not be all too appreciative of the fact that several pets before him carried the same name. Besides, tastes change. Just as the thought of eating broccoli turned your stomach when you were a child and now it's your favorite vegetable, that name you had chosen so long ago may now leave a bad taste in your mouth.

Parents find several different ways to begin the baby-naming process. To some, it is important to incorporate a family name, so this becomes their starting point. To others, religion is a major factor in choosing a name. Some prefer to seek out a meaning or virtue, while others simply want a name that sounds good. What it all boils down to is what is important to you. So, before you begin scouring these pages, making endless lists within our journaling prompts, and seeking the advice of others, be sure to determine what it is that you want from a name.

The following chapters offer advice, tips, and suggestions to help you maneuver the baby-naming maze for your future son, and hopefully have a little fun along the way. Follow a few simple guidelines, keep your mind open, save your humorous and cutesy titles for your pets, and your baby will have a name he is proud to hear, say, and write forever.

Above all, remember that the decision is yours and you are going to find the perfect fit for your little boy.

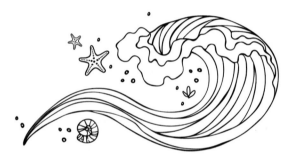

How to Choose
a Baby Name

P arents often find that the most challenging aspect
of choosing a name is knowing where to begin. Let's
face it: your kid has to live with the name you choose
forever. (Or at least until he's old enough to legally change
it himself.) To get going on your list, write down names
you have always liked. Was there someone in school
whose name you secretly wished you had? Did your favorite soap opera or sitcom have a character with a cool,
trendy name? Browse the names chapters of this book and
use the journaling prompts to jot down any that stand out
(or names you think of along the way). Perhaps you are
already receiving suggestions from friends and family.
Are there any that appeal to you? List all the names you
can think of that have caught your attention (in a good
way) and list any family names you'd consider using.

Once you have a few (or maybe a few sheets' worth),
consider the following attributes and see how each
measures up.

Popularity: Past, Present, and Future

Every year yields a new crop of trendy names that makes last year's list, well, outdated. While these fresh, fun names are fabulous and exciting, they also face the threat of being "so five minutes ago." Of course, there are those names that have always been and always will be popular; they're classic and chic, and they always make top-ten lists. They're the names that are trendy one minute, but still sound good thirty years from now. The key to giving your child a popular name that he or she can be proud of is to avoid trend traps altogether, such as movie-character names or TV-icon names that have a popularity shelf life of about six months. Often, a child named after a memorable television personality will always be linked with that person's TV character or personality traits.

One factor that makes a name popular is variation of spelling on a familiar or common name. While the new look might be pleasing to the eye, it might become a nuisance when you (and eventually your child) have to constantly correct others, telling them that Kristopher is spelled with a *K*, not a *C*. Similarly, if you're looking for an exceptionally rare name, you'll constantly be correcting both the spelling and the pronunciation.

At best, name trends give your child individualism. At worst, they ostracize him from a society of "regular" names. However, more and more parents are creating their own names or choosing from a more eclectic list of foreign names, vintage names, surnames, and place names. And since the unique-name pool is rapidly growing, chances are that your child's classmates will have unique names too.

The increasing popularity of foreign names allows parents to honor their families' cultures and give their children a sense of heritage. Irish, Scottish, and Welsh names are on the rise. Greek, Russian, and Italian names have more presence than they did years ago, as names like Nikos, Logan, Matteo, and Giovanni become more visible.

A recent revival of names like Charles, Willie, and George give a new perspective on some old favorites. While these names might seem classic or old-fashioned to us now, most of them were the trendy names of their time. During a period when a respectful tip of the hat was greeted by a graceful curtsy, these names reflected the chivalry and gentlemanly charm that made up society back then.

The use of surnames is another trend that seems to appear in cycles. Names like Carter, Sullivan, Kennedy, Taylor, Jackson, and Spencer can all be used for little boys. What's more, surnames can prove to be a convenient alternative to using the first name of a family member you'd like to honor.

And don't discount the nickname-as-name trend. Nowadays shorter nicknames like Finn and Dax are almost as popular as their longer counterparts, Finnegan and Daxton. So don't be shy if you want your boy's name to be short and sweet.

Meaning

A fun, creative, and often unique way to choose your child's name is to look for positive associations that come with the name. It also makes the naming process intentional and more special. If one of your favorite places is a wooded area where your family vacations once a year, look for names that have "trees" or "earthy" in their meanings. You can also look for names that reflect your favorite color, time of year, season, animal, art, character trait, and flower. If your favorite relative loves to visit Ireland every year, and you wish to honor him or her, choose an Irish name for your baby and use your relative's name for the middle name.

It's a good idea to look up the meaning of the names you've put on your list because the last thing you want is to frighten your child if he finds out his name means "unlucky in life." A name should evoke good feelings, positive thoughts, and pride. It should also be significant to you and your partner. Meanings are a way for your child to feel connected to you, to your family, and to life. Of course, if you like a name just because, that's okay too.

Family Names

Using family names to create your child's name is a wonderful way to pay tribute to loved ones. Additionally, if after five hours you're still staring at a blank piece of paper, jot down all the names of your family members, including grandparents, aunts, uncles, close cousins, or even close friends of the family.

What do you do if your late grandfather's name, Jerome, just isn't appealing to you, but you still want to include his name in your little boys'? The way around that is to us a variation instead, like Romey or Jerry. And if you'd love to honor your father, but Lawrence feels a bit too old-fashioned for your son's first name, how about adding it as his middle name or using a variation like Lars or Ren? The intent is still there, the name is more appealing, and the family is happy.

List some important family members and friends. Are there any names (or variations) here that you'd like to use for your little one?

....

....

....

....

....

....

....

....

....

Origin/Ancestry

Perhaps you want your son's name to indicate his heritage. After all, it's an important part of his identity, and connecting with it only adds to the richness of his character. Similarly, if you come from a particular religious background, you might want to explore that group of names too. If your family has been following a tradition for many generations, such as naming first-born children after saints, but you have a different name in mind, consider moving the traditional name to the middle. You'll make your family happy and still get to use the name you want.

If you and your partner come from different backgrounds, selecting one name from each to create the first and middle names is a great way to compromise. If you're still having issues over whose name goes first, make them both part of the first name and use a hyphen. As for whose name goes before the hyphen, pick one out of a hat and be done with it. Danny-Mack is a combination of the Hebrew Daniel and the Scottish Mack and has a trendy ring to it that any boy can love.

A family tree and history can be helpful resources when linking your baby's name with your heritage. For example, if your grandparents' ancestors come from a village in France where they operated a cheese business that had been passed on from generation to generation, the name Monterey would be fitting. Or, if there were many carpenters in the family, Cedar would be appropriate for your little boy.

Spelling and Pronunciation

While creative spellings and pronunciations of traditional names make a name unique, some parents can go a little crazy with it. The more difficult you make your child's name to spell and/or pronounce, the more annoying it becomes for them to constantly correct people.

Even if the name is as clear as Jeffrey, but spelled Jephree, your son will still have to spell it out every time someone writes it down because they will undoubtedly spell it traditionally. The following list provides examples of how a small change can have big impact on a name.

- Replace *i* or *e* with *y*: Chrystopher, Devyn, Eryk, Nathyn, Nicholys, Tymothy.
- Add an extra letter (silent *e*): Raymonde, Roberte, Ronalde, Shaye, Taylore.
- Replace *s* with *z*: Alexzander, Izaiah, Joziah, Julez.
- Add to or take away from double consonants: Antthony, Colin, Mathew, Robbert, Tobbias, Waren.
- Add a capital letter in the middle: DaKota, MacAuley, McKinley, LeBron, O'Reilly.

Stick to one change per name. Too many different styles make the name look like the parents were trying too hard to be different. Once you narrow your list of names down to the top contenders, play around with different spellings to see how each one looks on paper. Then, try the variants out on friends to see if they can easily recognize and pronounce the names.

Nicknames

As you narrow your search, anticipate any nicknames that could arise from both the name on its own as well as the first name and the last name together. It's inevitable that your child will receive several nicknames throughout his life (and some will have nothing to do with his name), so try to think of the ones that could have a negative effect. But don't let this scare you out of using the name you've fallen in love with. Unless they're obvious, most of the drawback names will probably never come up on the playground.

If you like a nickname and not its full name, consider using the nickname as the full name: Jamie instead of James, Alex instead of Alexander, Danny instead of Daniel. Or, you might consider using the full version of the name anyway to give your child the option of using it in a professional manner for résumés, interviews, and in titles like Dr. Daniel Green instead of Dr. Danny Green. Full names are formal and sound more professional. For that reason, people tend to enlist the services of professionals with more sophisticated names. See if you can tell the difference in the following sentence: *After having my taxes done by Daniel, I played soccer with Danny.* That's not to say that Danny wouldn't have prepared your taxes as accurately as Daniel would, or that Daniel wouldn't be fun to play soccer with. However, the names create different images in our minds because one is casual and the other is formal.

Full names tend to demand more respect and are more influential, whereas casual nicknames are associated with fun, relaxation, and lightheartedness. When Mom calls Danny by his full name, it usually means one thing—trouble. And when she calls him by his full first name and his middle name, he quickly learns that Mom means business!

15 Essentials for Finding and Choosing Names

The following are a few suggestions to help make the decision a little easier on you and your entire family.

Say the Names Out Loud

Often we think we like something, but then once we say it out loud, we realize it just isn't what we are looking for. This also works in the opposite way: you think you don't like a name until you say it out loud, and then realize it was exactly what you were looking for. Think of calling loudly for your children on the playground or to come in from playing outside for dinner. If you cringe when doing this, that name probably is not what you were looking for. You need to make sure you say all of your children's names together to see if they flow well. They shouldn't be overly similar or drastically dissimilar. Instead, find names that are harmonious without being singsongy.

Avoid Negative Namesakes

When choosing a name, steer clear of names that remind you of people you do not care for or that remind you of an ex-love. These names can only cause you problems in the future. You don't want to forever look at your son and think of that one Hunter from grade school who picked on you!

Say All Names Together

Say the name with not only the middle name, but with just the last name. We don't always use our children's middle names, but always use the last name, and if they don't sound right together or come out smoothly together, you need to keep looking.

Test Nicknames

Can your child's name hold up to the playground test? Are there ways that kids can turn the name into something awful that would crush your child's self-esteem and possibly brand him for life? Remember, kids can be cruel, especially siblings. Also make sure that your children won't have the same nicknames. This can happen if the names are too similar or if you use a feminine form of a masculine name for a girl and the masculine name itself for a boy.

Make It Meaningful

Your child's name should be something that makes you feel good. It should reflect qualities that you hope your child will someday possess. Be sure that every child's name is meaningful, not just one. For instance, little Calvin might become resentful if he finds out his name means "bald one" while his brother Aden's name means "handsome."

Keep in Mind Spelling and Pronunciations

Names that are difficult to spell and pronounce will be misspelled and mispronounced throughout the child's entire life. Also, keep in mind that using lengthy first names, middle names, and last names all together can be very difficult for a young child to learn to spell and say. An example would be Zachariah Emmanuel Klingele. The poor child would have to learn almost the entire alphabet to spell his name.

Be Creative

Try spelling names of things backward; many unique names can be discovered by doing this. For instance, if your name is Nora, perhaps Aron is the perfect name for your little boy. Also play around with dropping letters from established names to create new and unique names that you maybe hadn't thought of. For instance, Christopher can become Christoph, and Carlisle can become Lisle.

Use Maiden Names

A popular way of creating a baby name is by using the mother's maiden name or the maiden name of family members. Sullivan and Carter are good examples. This is also very popular for middle names as well.

Combine the Parents' Names

Another popular way of coming up with a baby name is by combining parts of the mother's and father's names. Brett and Everly might become Everett, or Samuel and Emma might be Emmanuel. This is done for both the first and middle names. However, if you do this, make sure you can also create a combined name for another child. Don't play favorites with names; it can affect the self-esteem of and relationship between siblings.

Try Out Different Spellings

You might like a name, but not care for the spelling, thinking it is perhaps too drab or too common. In being creative, anything goes. Sebastian might be Sebastyan; Isaiah might be Izaia; Aiden can become Aydon. But keep in mind that a child who has an unusual spelling will likely have to correct others over and over during his life.

Explore Genealogy

Another good way to find names is by exploring your family's genealogy. Do a family tree on both the baby's mother's side of the family and the baby's father's side, going back as far as you can. You might need some help from family members with this. Be sure to get the first, middle, and last names of everyone. Then go through these and look for names that stand out to you as something you would like to use. However, when doing this, keep in mind that some people are considered the black sheep of the family. If you settle on a name, be sure to get some background info on this person. You wouldn't want to name your baby something that reminds your mother of the person she most despises. This not only gives you some different names to choose from, but, if you keep it, would be a good gift for your children to have later. Kids love to hear about their ancestors. Again, consider choosing a name from your family tree for each child, not just one.

Ask for Suggestions

Talk to coworkers, neighbors, relatives, and friends. You don't have to use their opinions, but you will receive a ton of suggestions. Also ask them about people who have recently had babies and what those people named their children. This will not only give you name ideas, but will also tell you the names that are being used the most often.

Scour the Media

Consider names from books, television shows, movies, and celebrities. This can be a lot of fun, if you let it.

Consider the Classics

As a general rule of thumb, if your last name is unusual, it's a good idea to choose a more traditional first name. And if you have a common last name, choose a more distinctive first name. George Rothberry and Boomer Miller are some examples.

Look to Old-Fashioned Names

These names are making a comeback. They can be good choices because they have the ability to be both distinct and common. Names such as Walter and Clarence are both easily pronounced and spelled, but are not so common that there would be several in the same classroom.

Have Fun with It!

If you try to have fun and keep the task of choosing a name light, it will go much more smoothly. Making games out of the task is an easy way to take some of the stress off. Here are some game ideas that can be played with just a few people in the privacy of your home, or can be used at a baby shower or gender reveal to get guests to help with the process.

Find a piece of cardboard; it can even be an old cereal box opened up and laid out flat, plain side up. Make a game board similar to Monopoly or Candy Land, using baby names in the squares. You can use different coins or anything you choose for markers. Use a die and take turns rolling it to move around the board. Whoever gets to the end first gets to choose a name from the board to use. Play it four times, choosing four boy names to consider at the end.

Play Scrabble using the rule that you can only make baby names from the letters.

Take a piece of paper, and down one side put the letters of the alphabet, A–Z. Photocopy enough for each guest. Set a time limit and tell everyone to come up with a different or unique name for each letter. At the end, have guests read off the names they have, and any that match should be crossed off. The guest with the most names left wins a prize. The couple gets to keep these pages at the end to give them name ideas to choose from.

Take ten baby names; scramble the letters onto a piece of paper. Photocopy enough for each guest. Set a time limit and see who can come up with the most names using these letters. The couple keeps this at the end to refer to.

Write down the first and last name of the mother and father. Photocopy enough for each guest. Set a time limit and have each guest make names that begin with each letter of their names. Have the guests mark off any that match and see who has the most left at the end. The couple keeps this at the end to give them ideas.

Although this may seem like a long and extremely difficult task, keeping the spotlight on this joyous occasion will help. Try not to put so much pressure on yourself to have that exact and perfect name before the birth. This is not a task that should cause turmoil in the family, but joy.

Remember that naming your child is something that has been entrusted to you, by your baby.

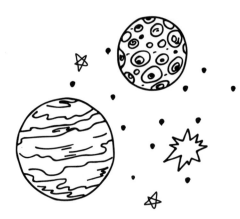

Names with Meaning

A name is more than just the sum of its letters— virtually every moniker is imbued with a particular meaning. Whether it's an attribute, personality trait, season, person, quality, place, or even product, the names you're thinking about have an inherent connection to other concepts. Discovering the meaning behind the names on your list is all part of the fun of naming your little boy. Since names can mean different things in different places and to different people, it's worth putting in some time to learn as much as you possibly can about the name you've chosen, both as a way to prevent negative associations and also as a source of inspiration.

Many parents-to-be cite meaning above all other attributes of a name as their primary inspiration for choosing it. In fact, deciding on a meaning first and then deciding on a name from the pool of contenders is a nice way to choose a firstborn's name, and possibly even other siblings' names down the road. There are two ways to approach this. You can start with an idea you love in a general way—say, for example, peace—and find out which names fit that concept, as Frederick, Soloman, and Galen do. Alternately, you can build from a more personal meaning that reflects your family specifically. If you're both army officers, for example, try Liam, Duncan, and Owen, all of which mean "protector" or "warrior."

Of course, meanings needn't always be hidden or obscure. Virtue names are an excellent example of this idea—names like Chance, Justice, and Honor certainly do put meaning front and center. There are also more spiritual names, like the classic Joseph and Ezekiel, or the more unique Asher and Tiras to evoke a specific meaning in your name choice. Wherever you find inspiration, try to choose a name that means something special to you and reflects positive attributes in general.

INSPIRATIONAL NAMES

Angel	Hope	Peace	True
Blessing	Justice	Prosper	Valor
Chance	Loyal	Revere	Wisdom
Genesis	Noble	Sincere	Worth
Honor	North	Trinity	Zen

Do you have any particular attributes (strength, wisdom, courage) that you'd like his name to highlight? List them here and see if you can discover some new options that mean the most to you!

....

....

....

....

....

....

....

....

....

....

....

....

....

....

....

....

....

....

....

....

BIBLICAL NAMES

Abel	Jacob	Luke	Solomon
Aron	Jedidah	Samson	
Benjamin	Joseph	Silas	

Variations on a Theme

Some groups of names go naturally together, and choosing from within a particular theme is a great way to narrow down the options or pick names for multiples or siblings. Try saint names like Casimir, Clement, and Eugene, or go more inspirational with Chance and True.

NAMES THAT MEAN "WISE"

Alden	Conroy	James	Tallis
Alfred	Emerson	Nathaniel	
Conaire	Henry	Ronald	

NAMES THAT MEAN "LIGHT"

Abner	Elior	Lucian	Zain
Anwar	Ivar	Oran	
Beacon	Kiran	Uri	

NAMES THAT MEAN "BLESSING" OR "GIFT" ··················

Barack	Hans	Nathan	Theodore
Benedict	Matteus	Niaz	
Doron	Matthew	Sean	

NAMES THAT MEAN "HANDSOME" ·······························

Aden	Cullen	Keane	Teague
Beau	Enver	Macallan	
Bellamy	Jamal	Paris	

NAMES THAT MEAN "STRONG" ·······························

Aaron	Charles	Magglio	Remo
Anders	Ethan	Nardo	Richard
Angus	Everett	Oscar	Steele
Arthur	Griffin	Pierce	Terrian
Cale	Kalmin	Quinlan	Valerian

ROYALTY NAMES ·······························

Duke	Kingston	Princeton	Royalty
Kensington	Knight	Reign	
King	Prince	Royal	

SAINT NAMES

Augustine	Clement	Maurice	Theobald
Benedict	Cyrus	Maximus	
Casimir	Gabriel	Simon	

NAMES FOR GREEK GODS

Adonis	Apollo	Erebus	Zeus
Aether	Ares	Eros	
Aion	Atlas	Hermes	

Unique Inspiration

There are people who like popular names, and there are people who don't. While one set of parents-to-be might choose the name Logan because it consistently ranks among the top ten boys' names, there are others who'd stay away from Logan for precisely that reason. For the latter group, there are plenty of other places to look for a unique name for your future son.

From specific sounds to unique categories, fantastic naming inspiration is everywhere! Look through some of your favorite books and movies—are there any characters or actors with unique names? What about a particular region—are you looking for something with a southern flair, or maybe some northeastern posh? What about playing around with spelling, finding a nickname that you love and using it as your boy's first name, or using some fantastic variants of popular favorites (Lucian for Lucas, Allister for Oliver)? The possibilities are endless.

Blending Favorites

Maybe you've narrowed it down to two choices and can't decide, or perhaps you simply want your little one's name to reflect both his parents: Samson and Grace became Grayson, Sebastian and Casey become Caspian, Rick and Alice become Alaric. It's a super-original way to make sure your little boy's name has the most meaning!

Here are some more places to look for unique names you may (or may not) find on any top 100 list:

SOUTHERN NAMES

Atkins	Garth	Jameson	Wiley
Beau	Gunnar	Landry	
Colt	Hank	Taylor	

PREPPY NAMES

Aldrich	Buckley	Hayes	Sterling
Ames	Connery	Kingsley	Thatcher
Anderson	Cornell	Montgomery	Whitaker
Briggs	Crosby	Pierce	Wilder
Brooks	Digby	Remington	Yates

CONSTELLATIONS

Canis	Crux	Orion	Sculptor
Centaurus	Dorado	Pavo	
Corvus	Draco	Phoenix	

NICKNAMES AS NAMES

Al	Dec	Jamie	Mav
Bash	Eli	Jax	Ollie
Beck	Finn	Jay	Rhett
Benny	Gray	Leo	Wes
Cam	Gus	Mac	Zach

COLORS

Ash	Brick	Jett	Sage
Auburn	Coal	Roux	
Azul	Gray	Rusty	

SHAKESPEAREAN NAMES

Claudius	Jaques	Peter	William
Henry	Lysander	Romeo	
Iago	Malcolm	Stephano	

NATURE NAMES

Ash	Elm	Hawke	Rio
Barrow	Everest	Hunter	River
Canyon	Fisher	Maverick	Talon
Cedar	Forrest	Ocean	Wilder
Colton	Fox	Rain	Wolfe

GRANDPA NAMES

Arthur	Felix	George	Walter
Edgar	Frances	Jeremiah	
Elmer	Frederick	Silas	

What are some of your favorite books? Are there any character names that you love?

....

....

....

....

....

....

....

....

....

LITERARY HEROES

Aeneas	Dorian	Holmes	Randle
Albus	Finn	Jay	Rhett
Atticus	Guy	Leopold	Richard
Caleb	Heathcliff	Marius	Robinson
Dean	Holden	Oliver	Tom

CHILDREN'S LIT NAMES

Calvin	Edmund	Max	Stuart
Caspian	Frank	Milo	Thomas
Charles	George	Percy	Willy
Wallace	Harold	Peter	
Charlie	Harry	Rowley	
Clifford	Klaus	Stanley	

FANDOM NAMES

Aragorn	Jean-Luc	Samwise	Tyrion
Gendry	Luke	Sirius	
Hans	Remus	Tardis	

CLASSIC NAMES

Alexander	Frederick	Julian	Vincent
Charles	Gabriel	Michael	
David	Geoffrey	Phillip	

FLAVORFUL NAMES

Asiago	Cayenne	Kale	Thyme
Basil	Colby	Kobe	
Caesar	Herb	Sage	

NAMES ON THE RISE

Colson	Kairo	Merrick	Wells
Gianluca	Kace	Nova	
Jaxxon	Ledger	Rowen	

NAMES THAT END IN -O

Aldo	Eliseo	Otto	Vito
Augusto	Marco	Silvio	
Cato	Oslo	Theo	

Top Alternatives to the Top 10

If you like an extremely popular name but wish it were more unique, here are some fresh alternatives you may find appealing.

Instead of Liam, try...

Callum	Declan	Lincoln
Cian	Leland	

Instead of Noah, try...

Jonah	Nico	Nolan
Milo	Noel	

Instead of William, try...

Elias	Wiley	Wilson
Liam	Willem	

Instead of James, try...

Jamie	Jayce	Miles
Jay	Jonas	

Instead of Logan, try...

Keagon	Lawson	Owen
Lachlan	Lennon	

Instead of Benjamin, try...

Bartholomew	Benji	Reuben
Benedict	James	

Instead of Mason, try...

Asa	Kason	Maximus
Emerson	Maddox	

Instead of Elijah, try...

Eli	Eliha	Josiah
Elias	Ezra	

Instead of Oliver, try...

Archer	Leo	Olivier
Elliot	Oli	

Instead of Jacob, try...

Caleb	Jake	Joshua
Jackson	Jonah	

Anything that sparked your interest? What are some of your favorite trendy names? List them here.

....

....

....

....

....

....

....

....

....

Famous Influence

Certain names evoke certain feelings in people, which is often why we turn to some of our favorite, and most famous, friends for naming inspiration. Whether it be your favorite sports star, a powerful male scientist, an exemplary author, or the celebrity or singer you look up to the most, famous names are often a great place to start when you're looking to name your future son.

However, one thing to keep in mind: whether fictional or not, certain names are forever embedded in our psyche as having very specific character traits or legacies. You'll need to remember these associations when creating the name that your child will live with for the rest of his life. Like it or not, Kobe, Prince, Barack, Abraham, Martin Luther, and Elvis will always bring to mind the personalities they're most often associated with. If you adore the legacy these names have left behind, then forge ahead!

Here are some famous male powerhouses to browse through.

ACTIVISTS

Booker	Frederick	Martin	Thurgood
Cesar	Mahatma	Nelson	
Charlton	Malcolm	Paul	

COUNTRY SINGERS

Cole	Garth	Jason	Willie
Conway	Hank	Travis	
Eric	Kenny	Waylon	

CLASSIC MOVIE STARS

Alfred	Clint	James	Montgomery
Burt	Fred	John	Orson
Cary	Gene	Laurence	Robert
Charles	Gregory	Marlon	Sidney
Clark	Humphrey	Mickey	Spencer

POP STAR NAMES

Bruno	Harry	Prince	Zayn
David	Justin	Shawn	
Elvis	Michael	Usher	

FASHION DESIGNERS

Alexander	Giorgio	Marc	Zac
Christian	Jimmy	Oscar	
Emilio	Karl	Riccardo	

PRESIDENTIAL NAMES

Carter	James	McKinley	Taylor
Hayes	Kennedy	Monroe	
Jackson	Madison	Reagan	

Art Attack

Scour your favorite movies, books, and music for ideas. Jazz fans may want to choose Miles or Billie; art lovers, Pablo or Vincent; cinema connoisseurs, Steven or Quentin.

ARTISTS

Andy	Jackson	Salvador
Claude	Johannes	Vincent
Edvard	Leonardo	
Georges	Pablo	

COMEDIANS

Andy	Eddie	Robin	Woody
Aziz	Jerry	Rodney	
Chris	Richard	Steve	

POETS

Allen	Dante	Seamus	Yeats
Auden	Eliot	Sherman	
Byron	Langston	Walt	

SPORTS LEGENDS

Babe	Michael	Roger	Wayne
Jackie	Muhammad	Tiger	
Lionel	Peyton	Usain	

SCIENTISTS

Albert	Galileo	Nikola	Thomas
Alexander	Isaac	Sigmund	
Charles	Niels	Stephen	

CELEBRITY NAMES

Bradley	Dwayne	Hugh	Russell
Clint	Harrison	Leonardo	
Denzel	Heath	Morgan	

What are some of your favorite famous inspirations? Any names you may want to adopt for your own little one?

....

....

....

....

....

....

....

....

....

....

....

....

....

....

....

....

....

....

....

....

....

Celebrity Baby Names A–Z

Our society is fascinated with the names celebrities choose for their children. Any new celebrity birth instantly makes headlines. So, whether you're looking for inspiration or you're just curious, here's an alphabetical listing of baby names and the celebrities who chose them.

Alastair Wallace

Rod Stewart and Penny Lancaster

Alfie

Gary Oldman and Lesley Manville

Apollo Bowie Flynn

Gavin Rossdale and Gwen Stefani

Archibald William Emerson

Will Arnett and Amy Poehler

Arpad Flynn Alexander

Arpad Busson and Elle MacPherson

Arthur Saint

Jason Bleick and Selma Blair

Ashe Olsen

Seth Meyers and Alexi Ashe

Augustus Alexis

David Arquette and Christina Arquette

Axel

Will Ferrell and Viveca Paulin

Axel Strahl

Seth Meyers and Alexi Ashe

Bear Blu

Christopher Jarecki and Alicia Silverstone

Beaumont Gino

Jordan Peele and Chelsea Peretti

Beckett Richard

Michael Phelps and Nicole Johnson

Bingham Hawn

Matthew Bellamy and Kate Hudson

Bodhi Ransom

Brian Austin Green and Megan Fox

Boomer Robert

Michael Phelps and Nicole Johnson

Brendan Joseph

Mark Wahlberg and Rhea Durham

Bronx Mowgli

Pete Wentz and Ashlee Simpson

Brooklyn Joseph

David Beckham and Victoria Beckham

Bryce Maximus

LeBron James and Savannah James

Caleb Kelechi

Nnamdi Asomugha and Kerry Washington

Camden Jack

Jay Cutler and Kristin Cavallari

Canon Wardell Jack

Stephen Curry and Ayesha Curry

Cash Alexander

Wade Allen and Annabeth Gish

Caspar Matthew

Matthew Vaughn and Claudia Schiffer

Charlie Axel

Tiger Woods and Elin Nordegren

Charlie Wolf

Jacob Pechenik and Zooey Deschanel

Crew

Chip Gaines and Joanna Gaines

Darby Galen

Patrick Dempsey and Jillian Dempsey

Deacon Reese

Ryan Phillippe and Reese Witherspoon

Denim Cole

Keri Lewis and Toni Braxton

Dimitri Portwood

Ashton Kutcher and Mila Kunis

Donovan Rory

Noel Gallagher and Sara MacDonald

Duncan Zowie Haywood Jones

David Bowie and Angela Bowie

Duke

Diane Keaton

Edward Duke

Bill Rancic and Giuliana Rancic

Elias

Michael Bublé and Luisana Lopilato

Emet Kuli

Roey Hershkovitz and Lisa Loeb

Ennis Howard

Jesse Plemons and Kirsten Dunst

Exton Elias

Robert Downey Jr. and Susan Downey

Finn

Owen Wilson and Caroline Lindqvist

Forrest Bradley

Eric Decker and Jessie James Decker

Francisco

Lin-Manuel Miranda and Vanessa Nadal

Freddie Reign

Louis Tomlinson and Briana Jungwirth

Gable Ness

Kevin Nealon and Susan Yeagley

Genesis Ali Dean

Swizz Beatz and Alicia Keys

George Alexander Louis

The Duke and Duchess of Cambridge

Gideon Scott

Neil Patrick Harris and David Burtka

Griffin Thomas

Joey McIntyre and Barrett Williams

Gulliver Flynn

Gary Oldman and Donya Fiorentino

Hal Auden

Benedict Cumberbatch and Sophie Hunter

Hawkins

Tony Romo and Candice Crawford

Hayes Logan

Kevin Costner and Christine Baumgartner

Henry Chance

Darren Aronofsky and Rachel Weisz

Holden Fletcher

Brendan Fraser and Afton Smith

Homer James Jigme

Richard Gere and Carey Lowell

Hopper Jack

Sean Penn and Robin Wright

Hud

John Mellencamp and Elaine Irwin

Hugo Wilson

Josh Dallas and Ginnifer Goodwin

Ignatius Martin

Andrew Upton and Cate Blanchett

Indio

Robert Downey Jr. and Deborah Falconer

Isaiah Akin

Isaiah Washington and Jenisa Marie Washington

Iver Eames

James Conran and Coco Rocha

Jack Oscar

Jason Statham and Rosie Huntington-Whiteley

Jaden

Will Smith and Jada Pinkett Smith

Jagger Joseph Blue

Jason Goldberg and Soleil Moon Frye

Jameson Moon

Carey Hart and Pink

Jasper Warren

Brad Paisley and Kimberly Paisley

Jayden James

Kevin Federline and Britney Spears

Johan Riley Fyodor Taiwo

Seal and Heidi Klum

John Edward Thomas

Tom Brady and Bridget Moynahan

Jonas Rocket

Tom DeLonge and Jennifer DeLonge

Journey River

Brian Austin Green and Megan Fox

Julian Fuego

Robin Thicke and Paula Patton

Justin

Andie MacDowell and Paul Qualley

Kal-El Coppola

Nicolas Cage and Alice Kim

Kase Townes

Ty Murray and Jewel

Keen

Mark Ruffalo and Sunrise Coigney

Kenzo Kash

Kevin Hart and Eniko Parrish

Kingston James McGregor

Gavin Rossdale and Gwen Stefani

Knox Léon

Brad Pitt and Angelina Jolie

Laird Vonne

Sharon Stone

Levi Alves

Matthew McConaughey and Camila Alves

Liam James

William Tell and Lauren Conrad

Louis Bardo

Sandra Bullock

Lucian

Steve Buscemi and Jo Andres

Maceo Robert

Olivier Martinez and Halle Berry

Maddox Chivan Thornton

Brad Pitt and Angelina Jolie

Magnus Mitchell

Max Handelman and Elizabeth Banks

Mason Dash

Scott Disick and Kourtney Kardashian

Mateo Bravery

Benjamin Bratt and Talisa Soto

Miles Theodore Stephens

John Legend and Chrissy Teigen

Moses Bruce Anthony

Chris Martin and Gwyneth Paltrow

Nathan Thomas

Jon Stewart and Tracey McShane

Nayib

Emilio Estefan and Gloria Estefan

Ocean Alexander

Forest Whitaker and Raye Dowell

Oliver Philip

Fred Savage and Jennifer Stone

Orion Christopher

Chris Noth and Tara Wilson

Otis Tobias

Tobey Maguire and Jennifer Meyer

Otto

Christian Hebel and Rachael Harris

Pax Thien

Brad Pitt and Angelina Jolie

Phinnaeus Walter

Daniel Moder and Julia Roberts

Presley Walker

Rande Gerber and Cindy Crawford

Prince Michael

Michael Jackson and Debbie Rowe

Quinn Kelly

Sharon Stone

Racer Maximilliano

Robert Rodriguez and Elizabeth Avellan

Rebel Antonio

Robert Rodriguez and Elizabeth Avellan

Reign Aston

Scott Disick and Kourtney Kardashian

Remington Alexander

Brandon Blackstock and Kelly Clarkson

River Russell

Shane Deary and Keri Russell

Roman Alexander-Raj

Ne-Yo and Crystal Renay

Ronan Cal

Daniel Day-Lewis and Rebecca Miller

Ryder Falcon

Rodney Atkins and Rose Falcon Atkins

Samuel Kai

Liev Schreiber and Naomi Watts

Sean Preston

Kevin Federline and Britney Spears

Sebastian Piers

Ryan Piers Williams and America Ferrera

Shepherd Kellen

Jerry Seinfeld and Jessica Seinfeld

Sir

Jay-Z and Beyoncé

Slater Josiah

Courtney B. Vance and Angela Bassett

Sparrow James Midnight

Joel Madden and Nicole Richie

Sullivan Patrick

Patrick Dempsey and Jillian Dempsey

Tennessee James

Jim Toth and Reese Witherspoon

Tennyson

Russell Crowe and Danielle Spencer

Titan Jewell

Tim Weatherspoon and Kelly Rowland

Truman Theodore

Tom Hanks and Rita Wilson

Valentino

Ricky Martin

Walker Nathaniel

Taye Diggs and Idina Menzel

Weston Lee

Lee Kirk and Jenna Fischer

Wilder Brooks

Oliver Hudson and Erinn Bartlett

William Huckleberry

Brad Paisley and Kimberly Williams-Paisley

Xander Dane

January Jones

York

Erik Asla and Tyra Banks

Zander Ryan

Billy McKnight and Mindy McCready

Zephyr

Robby Benson and Karla DeVito

Zion Malachi Airamis

Dwyane Wade and Siohvaughn Funches

Unisex Favorites

Unisex names have been around for ages, but they are just now pushing their way to the forefront of popularity. This could be due to the fact that there are more parents who want to strip their children of gender restraints. For instance, when the résumé of Jordan Smith crosses the HR director's desk, there will be no way for him or her to tell whether Jordan is a man or woman, and therefore all gender bias has been erased. Jordan will have to secure that interview on merit alone. On the other hand, some parents choose unisex names because of the associations they carry. For instance, parents may want their son's name to embody grace and beauty; after all, he's going to be strong and tough already, so why would he need a classically masculine name to reiterate that? Choosing a more feminine or gender-neutral name may accomplish this.

Some parents want to give their children names that are a bit unusual, those that will set their children apart in the sea of Jacobs and Barrys. Unisex names break away from traditional masculine names, adding to the pot a variety of choices that will make the classroom roster a bit more colorful. There is also a wide variety of meanings to choose from. Whether you are looking for a name from nature, a place name, a name meaning "strength," a name meaning "beauty," or a name meaning "benevolence," you can find it in the list of unisex names available today.

A unisex name is one that can be used for either gender. Lots of names are popular for both boys and girls, but they're generally more popular for one gender than the other. Historically, most unisex names began as boys' names but for one reason or another began to appeal to parents of girls. Once it becomes common for girls to take on these names, they become unisex, though sometimes, the pattern works in reverse. Names such as Lindsay and Florence are true unisex names, as they have their roots in masculinity, but they have been so predominantly used for girls that they are considered to be part of the girls' names and are no longer often seen as an option for boys. The following is a list of the top unisex names—names that appear in both the boys' and girls' top 1,000 names as compiled by the Social Security Administration. We've broken these up by how predominately they are used by girls versus boys.

Spelling Matters!

If you're going to choose...

Cameron/Camryn/Kamryn: Cameron is the more popular choices for boys, Camryn and Kamryn for girls

Skylar/Skyler: Skyler is more popular for boys, while Skylar wins for girls

Jordan/Jordyn: Jordan is more popular for boys, Jordyn for girls

NEARLY EQUAL

Charlie	Landry	River	Skyler
Justice	Oakley	Rowan	

MORE POPULAR FOR BOYS

Amari	Dallas	Jordan	Remy
Angel	Dylan	Kai	Rory
Ari	Elliot	Lennox	Royal
Blake	Ellis	Logan	Ryan
Cameron	Hayden	Micah	Rylan
Carter	Hunter	Parker	Sawyer
Casey	Jayden	Phoenix	Zion

OTHER OPTIONS

Alexis	Finley	London	Reese
Ariel	Harley	Lyric	Riley
Avery	Harper	Marley	Sage
Dakota	Jamie	Morgan	Skylar
Eden	Jessie	Nova	Sutton
Emerson	Kendall	Payton	Tatum
Emery	Leighton	Peyton	Taylor
Emory	Lennon	Quinn	

UNDER THE RADAR

Arlo	Frankie	Jules	Wyatt
Brett	Gray	Monroe	
Delta	James	Stevie	

What are some unisex names you love? Did you just find the perfect gender-neutral option for your little boy?

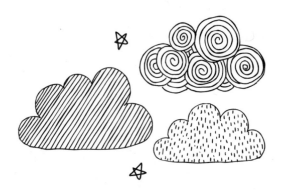

Around the World

In this era of globalization, baby-name trends are not immune to worldwide influence. While many parents choose to honor their roots by selecting a name from their own ethnic background, it appears that having a familial connection to an ethnicity is not a prerequisite for choosing a name from that ethnicity. This is actually not a brand-new trend; it has happened before that one ethnicity's names take on a mainstream popularity for a period of time. For instance, names of Hispanic origin became popular in the sixties, leading to the rise in popularity of names like Juan among non-Hispanics. However, never before has the average parent had access to such a wide variety of names. Here are just a few places you can look when naming your new little one.

Celtic Names

Americans specifically have long held a fascination with Celtic culture. Recently, this interest has grown in magnitude and strength, helped along by the rising popularity of Celtic literature, music, and dance, and the fact that so many Americans trace their roots back to the Celtic strongholds of Wales, England, Ireland, and Scotland. Many of these names have grown in popularity so much that they have lost the slightly odd, new feeling many names from other countries have. Many new Celtic names have been increasingly breaking into the ranks of common American baby names.

From Ireland, some of the more popular boys' names are Aidan, Colin, Connor, Kyan, Murray, Quinn, and Teagan.

Scotland has contributed many names from last names, but Scottish first names are also popular choices for American parents. Scottish boys' names include Alasdair, Blair, Calum, Fraser, Euan, Hamish, Lauchlan, and Malcolm.

Wales is also a prominent source for Celtic names today. Some increasingly popular Welsh names for boys are Ioan, Rhys, Dafydd (David), Dewey, Gareth, Quinn, and Maddock.

Other Celtic peoples, such as the Bretons and Cornish, also contribute to the Celtic naming trend but not yet on the scale that the others do. Here's a look at some of our Celtic favorites.

POPULAR NAMES IN IRELAND

Charlie	Conor	Jack	Sean
Cian	Darragh	Oisin	
Cillian	Fionn	Patrick	

POPULAR NAMES IN SCOTLAND

Alfie	Euan	Murray	Rory
Blair	Finlay	Oliver	
Callum	Harris	Rhys	

POPULAR NAMES IN WALES

Aeron	Carwyn	Jac	Owen
Aled	Dylan	Oliver	
Archie	Hari	Osian	

British Names

One can argue that Britain and the United States draw from a nearly similar name pool. However, certain names are used in each country that are rarely used in the other. With the success of many British authors, notably J. K. Rowling (*Harry Potter*) and Helen Fielding (*Bridget*

Jones), and British films and television programs in the United States, some of these uniquely British names have been working their way into American popular consciousness and thus into baby-naming trends as well.

POPULAR NAMES IN ENGLAND

Albert	Harrison	Louie	William
Arlo	Hugo	Oscar	
George	Lewis	Teddy	

African Names

Obviously, Africa is a continent of many nations and peoples and accordingly a source of great variety of names and naming customs. In recent times, many Americans of African descent have looked to Africa for names that represent their history and culture and their pride therein. However, African names have also been shown to appeal to a broader spectrum of the public. There is a wide variety of sources for traditional African names, including information about the origin and meanings. Since there are so many distinct cultures and peoples in Africa, we will just list a few of the more well-known names in America for boys: Abdul, Farid, Maalik, Tahir, and Tan.

POPULAR NAMES IN NIGERIA

Abdulai	Faruq	Ismail	Umar
Adamu	Ibrahim	Jidda	
Ali	Isa	Musa	

POPULAR NAMES IN SOUTH AFRICA

Amogelang	Enzokuhle	Lubanzi	Siyabonga
Bandile	Junior	Melokuhle	
Bokamoso	Lethabo	Mpho	

What is your own heritage? Are there any names from that country or culture that have always stuck out to you?

....

....

....

....

....

....

....

....

....

....

Popular Names Around the World

Let's take a look at some other popular favorites from across the globe.

POPULAR NAMES IN AUSTRALIA

Archer	Harvey	Levi	Riley
Cooper	Hudson	Mason	
Harry	Lachlan	Noah	

POPULAR NAMES IN BRAZIL

Davi	Felipe	Miguel	Thiago
Eduardo	Guilherme	Pedro	
Enzo	Gustavo	Pietro	

POPULAR NAMES IN CANADA

Aiden	Ethan	Jackson	Nathan
Benjamin	Grayson	Lincoln	
Carter	Jack	Logan	

POPULAR NAMES IN FRANCE

Antoine	Gabriel	Pierre	Theo
Clement	Jules	Quentin	
Florian	Leo	Raphaël	

POPULAR NAMES IN GERMANY ··

Anton	Henri	Max	Oskar
Elias	Leon	Maximilian	
Emil	Luka	Moritz	

POPULAR NAMES IN ISRAEL ··

Abraham	Itai	Noam	Yair
Ariel	Joseph	Omer	
Eitan	Lavi	Uri	

POPULAR NAMES IN ITALY ··

Davide	Giovanni	Luca	Stefano
Diego	Giuseppe	Marco	
Francesco	Lorenzo	Mattia	

POPULAR NAMES IN JAPAN ··

Arata	Hinata	Ren	Yuuma
Asahi	Hiroto	Sou	
Haruto	Isuki	Yuu	

POPULAR NAMES IN NEW ZEALAND ··

Arlo	Cohen	Hudson	Toby
Beau	Ezra	James	
Bodhi	Felix	Nixon	

POPULAR NAMES IN NORWAY

Aksel	Isak	Magnus	Tobias
Filip	Jakob	Mathias	
Håkon	Ludvig	Olav	

POPULAR NAMES IN SPAIN

Adrian	Daniel	Hugo	Pablo
Alejandro	David	Javier	
Alvaro	Diego	Mario	

POPULAR NAMES IN SWEDEN

Anders	Johan	Mikael	Per
Erik	Karl	Nils	
Jan	Lars	Olof	

POPULAR NAMES IN TURKEY

Ahmet	Eymen	Miraç	Yusuf
Berat	Hamza	Mustafa	
Emir	Mehmet	Ömer	

Classic Options

Since the American people are composed of people from many different countries, we can expect a wide variety of names to appear on the landscape, many of which will have broad appeal. Classic names from countries like France (Lucien and Noe for boys), Germany, and Italy have also increased in popularity. Middle Eastern, Indian, Chinese, Japanese, and other countries and cultures are contributing names on an ever-increasing basis due to the "shrinking globe." Hispanic names, some of which are already quite common, are also increasing in frequency of use. Russian names such as Andrei, Adrian, and Dimitri are being used. The names Misha and Nikita are being given as names for female children, even though in Russian they are traditionally male names (Misha being a diminutive for Mikhail).

For parents who are looking into ethnic names, there are numerous websites and books that cover each country or region and give meanings and origins of the names as well. It is particularly important for parents who have little or no background with a certain country or group to look into the meanings and associations with certain names.

AFRICAN NAMES

Abasi	Kami	Mazi	Zira
Adom	Jafari	Mukasa	
Hanif	Juman	Obinna	

AFRICAN AMERICAN NAMES

Antwon	Denzel	Jaylen	Rashaun
Barack	Deshawn	Jeremiah	Shaquille
Cameron	Jabari	Keshawn	Tyrell
Clive	Jaden	Malik	Tyrone
Darnell	Jaleel	Miles	Zion

ARABIC NAMES

Ali	Jaspar	Nasir	Tamir
Ayaan	Khalil	Omari	
Amir	Malik	Saleem	

ASIAN NAMES

Aki	Jin	Naoki	Zian
Bourey	Kaede	Raiden	
Dara	Kiri	Sanjay	

DUTCH NAMES

Daley	Morris	Senn	Willem
Floris	Niek	Siem	
Hidde	Noud	Stef	

FRENCH NAMES

Alexandre	Françoise	Léon	Quentin
Antoine	Gabin	Loïc	Sébastian
Augustin	Gaspard	Maël	Timothée
Clement	Jacques	Marceau	Tristan
Étienne	Jules	Pierre	Valentine

GERMAN NAMES

Christian	Hans	Niklas	Wilhelm
Dieter	Jannik	Otto	
Ernst	Klaus	Werner	

GREEK NAMES

Adrian	Homer	Neo	Spiro
Constantine	Icarus	Rastus	
Corban	Kristo	Santos	

IRISH NAMES

Brady	Finnegan	Niall	Tiernan
Cormac	Keegan	Quinn	
Donnelly	Killian	Rohan	

ITALIAN NAMES

Alba	Dante	Matteo	Sergio
Ambrosi	Emanuele	Niccolo	
Armond	Giacomo	Rocco	

POLISH NAMES

Borys	Igor	Marek	Witold
Fabian	Krystian	Tomasz	
Filip	Leon	Tymon	

ROMAN NAMES

Atticus	Felix	Maximus	Rufus
Augustus	Julius	Philo	
Cato	Magnus	Remus	

SCOTTISH NAMES

Adair	Gregor	Lachlan	Stuart
Duncan	Hamish	Macaulay	
Fergus	Iain	Padraig	

SPANISH NAMES

Alvaro	Dario	Manuel	Santiago
Antonio	Hector	Miguel	
Carlos	Luis	Rafael	

WELSH NAMES ··

Alwyn	Dai	Gruffydd	Wynn
Bran	Emrick	Rhain	
Dafydd	Ewan	Rhys	

Are there any names from around the world that you find striking? Make a list of some of your favorites and where they are from. Is there any country that you're particularly drawn to?

....

....

....

....

....

....

....

....

....

....

....

....

....

....

Uniquely American

Americans are a creative people, not bound by tradition and rules. These qualities are expressed in naming as well. Early Americans happily used adjectives describing desired qualities for their children, including Patience, Temperance, Makepeace, and Prudence. Many of these names are making a comeback, along with Hope, Faith, Joy, and Peace. Many popular American names come from American Indian names, words, and tribes (Cheyenne, Dakota, Cherokee). However, parents seeking to name their children one of these names should do their research. There is a lot of folklore surrounding names that is inaccurate, and some names may have special status for American Indians, where naming a child with that name may be disrespectful.

NATIVE AMERICAN TRIBAL NAMES

Apache	Comanche	Seminole	Shoshone
Cherokee	Dakota	Seneca	
Cheyenne	Navajo	Shawnee	

PATRIOTIC NAMES

America	July	Lincoln
Ellis	Justice	Spirit
Frances	Knox	
Glory	Liberty	

Global Village

It may seem an unlikely approach, but maps, globes, and even road atlases are an amazing source of onomatological wealth. Look to street names, towns, rivers, mountains, and far-off places to yield a rich variety of meanings and sounds. If it's a place you happen to know and love, all the better.

Place Names

Maps have long provided inspiration in the naming of children, whether because the locale had a particular significance to the parents, or just because they liked the way it sounded. Many children share their names with cities, states, countries, and regions.

Celebrities appear to be spearheading the revival of this trend; Madonna named her daughter Lourdes; David Beckham named his son Brooklyn; and then there is Paris Hilton. Names like China and India have been around for a while. Some state names have become quite common, like Virginia, Georgia, and Carolina. Other states are now starting to appear on birth certificates, like Dakota, Indiana, and Montana. Cities are also inspiring parents: Savannah, Austin, Houston, Atlanta, and Phoenix. Even ancient lands and cities, such as Troy and Atlantis, are popular names. Country names often used include Israel,

Cuba, Kenya, and Jordan. Many of these names are considered unisex; some are primarily one or the other depending on whether the sound of the name is more feminine or masculine to the parents.

PLACE NAMES

Aspen	Caspian	Kashmir	Raleigh
Austin	Chandler	Lawrence	Scotland
Bronx	Denver	Morocco	Troy
Brooklyn	Euston	Paris	York
Cairo	Indio	Phoenix	Zaire

Top Names
Throughout History

Names, like fashion, go in and out of vogue. Each time period seems to have a certain naming style that defines it. Currently, the Todds, Joels, and Brians of the 1990s have been replaced with Liams, Logans, and Noahs. So what exactly are the hottest names from the past? Here's a look at the top names from each decade (and some new rising favorites):

MOST POPULAR OF THE 1940S

Charles	James	Robert	William
David	John	Ronald	
Donald	Richard	Thomas	

MOST POPULAR OF THE 1950S

Charles	James	Richard	William
David	John	Robert	
Gary	Michael	Thomas	

MOST POPULAR OF THE 1960S ·····························

David	Mark	Robert	William
James	Michael	Steven	
John	Richard	Thomas	

MOST POPULAR OF THE 1970S ·····························

Brian	James	Michael	William
Christopher	John	Richard	
David	Mark	Robert	

MOST POPULAR OF THE 1980S ·····························

Christopher	Jason	Joshua	Robert
David	John	Matthew	
James	Joseph	Michael	

MOST POPULAR OF THE 1990S ·····························

Andrew	David	Joshua	Michael
Christopher	James	Justin	
Daniel	Joseph	Matthew	

MOST POPULAR OF 2000S ·····························

Andrew	Jacob	Matthew	Tyler
Christopher	Joseph	Michael	
Daniel	Joshua	Nicholas	

MOST POPULAR OF 2010

Aiden	Daniel	Jayden	William
Alexander	Ethan	Michael	
Anthony	Jacob	Noah	

MOST POPULAR NAMES OF 2015

Alexander	Jacob	Mason	William
Benjamin	James	Michael	
Ethan	Liam	Noah	

MOST POPULAR NAMES EXPECTED IN 2020

Aiden	Jackson	Mason	Oliver
Alexander	James	Michael	
Elijah	Liam	Noah	

NAMES ON THE RISE

Ayan	Gatlin	Khari	Nova
Bjorn	Gordon	Koa	Ridge
Briar	Juelz	Ledger	Shepard
Colson	Kannon	Marcelo	Wesson
Frankie	Kashton	Musa	Yadiel

NAMES UNDER THE RADAR ··

Alaric	Ezequiel	Leland	Sage
Axton	Gianni	Mack	Tadeo
Bodhi	Jordy	Otto	Winston
Colt	Keanu	Randall	Yousef
Dax	Kyree	Rey	Zayn

Names from A to Z

Do you want your future son's name to start with the same letter as yours? Or maybe you want your little boy's name to start with the most (or least) popular letter of the alphabet? You may find it surprising, but recently only eleven of the top 1,000 boy baby names start with an O: Oakley, Odin, Oliver, Omar, Omari, Orion, Orlando, Oscar, Otis, Otto, and Owen. At the same time, you probably won't find it as surprising that the most popular letter that boys' names start with is A (97 of the top 1,000), with J as a close second with 95 names. Take a look at some other names for each letter:

A NAMES

Abel	Alessandro	Anderson	Axel
Adriel	Alvaro	Andrew	
Alan	Amos	Ari	

B NAMES

Beckett	Blaine	Briggs	Byron
Bentley	Braden	Brodie	
Bishop	Brett	Brooks	

C NAMES

Cain	Carter	Charles	Cristian
Callan	Cassius	Cole	
Cameron	Cedric	Corey	

D NAMES

Dallas	David	Declan	Drake
Damian	Dawson	Desmond	
Darrell	Deacon	Dominick	

E NAMES

Easton	Ellis	Enrique	Ezekiel
Edison	Emanuel	Enzo	
Eliseo	Emmett	Ethan	

F NAMES

Fabian	Fletcher	Foster	Frederick
Felix	Flynn	Francis	
Finnley	Forrest	Franklin	

G NAMES

Gabriel	Gianni	Gregory	Gustavo
Gerald	Gideon	Greyson	
Giancarlo	Graham	Gunner	

H NAMES

Hamza	Harrison	Hendrix	Hugo
Harlen	Hassan	Howard	
Harper	Hayden	Hudson	

I NAMES

Ian	Ira	Ishaan	Izaiah
Ibrahim	Isaac	Israel	
Iker	Isaias	Ivan	

J NAMES

Jace	Jameson	Joaquin	Julius
Jagger	Jasper	Joel	
Jaiden	Jensen	Jordy	

K NAMES

Kai	Kareem	Kian	Kyrie
Kamryn	Keith	Kody	
Kannon	Kendrick	Kyle	

L NAMES

Lamar	Lennon	Lionel	Lyle
Landry	Leonard	Louie	
Lawson	Leroy	Lucca	

M NAMES

Maddox	Maurice	Micah	Morgan
Malachi	Maximo	Miles	
Marcel	Memphis	Moises	

N NAMES

Nash	Nehemiah	Nicholas	Nova
Nasir	Neil	Nico	
Nathan	Nelson	Noel	

O NAMES

Oakley	Omar	Oscar	Owen
Odin	Orion	Otis	
Oliver	Orlando	Otto	

P NAMES

Parker	Peter	Phoenix	Princeton
Paul	Peyton	Porter	
Paxton	Phillip	Preston	

Q NAMES

Qeleigh	Quierian	Quincy	Quirien
Quade	Quinby	Quinn	
Quentin	Quincie	Quinton	

R NAMES

Raiden	Reed	Rhys	Russell
Ramon	Reginald	Riley	
Ray	Remington	Rodney	

S NAMES

Salvador	Sawyer	Sonny	Sylas
Sam	Scott	Stephen	
Santos	Simeon	Sutton	

T NAMES

Talon	Thaddeus	Tony	Tucker
Tanner	Thatcher	Tripp	
Terrence	Tobias	Tristan	

U NAMES

Ugo	Ulises	Umberto	Uriel
Ulfred	Ulmer	Uriah	
Uli	Ulric	Urian	

V NAMES

Valentin	Vance	Victor	Vivaan
Valentino	Vaughn	Vihaan	
Van	Vicente	Vincent	

W NAMES

Wade	Wells	Wilder	Wyatt
Warren	Wesson	William	
Waylon	Weston	Winston	

X NAMES

Xackery	Xavier	Xeno	Xuan
Xander	Xavi	Xenos	
Xandros	Xavion	Xidorn	

Y NAMES

Yadiel	Yareli	Yorick	Yusuf
Yahir	Yehuda	Yosef	
Yahya	Yisroel	Yousef	

Z NAMES ···

Zachariah	Zaire	Zayn	Zion
Zahir	Zander	Zechariah	
Zaid	Zayden	Zeke	

What does your name start with? Your partner's? List some options for each letter below.

....

....

....

....

....

....

....

....

....

....

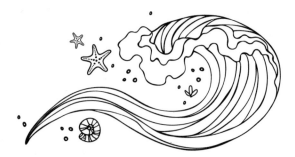

700 BOYS' NAMES

A

Aaden (Irish) Form of Aidan, meaning "a fiery young man" *Adan, Aden*

Aaron (Hebrew) One who is exalted; from the mountain of strength *Aaran, Aaren, Aarin, Aaro, Aaronas, Aaronn, Aarron, Aaryn, Eron, Aron, Eran*

Abdul (Arabic) A servant of God *Abdal, Abdall, Abdalla, Abdallah, Abdel, Abdell, Abdella, Abdellah*

Abel (Hebrew) The life force, breath *Abele, Abell, Abelson, Able, Avel, Avele*

Abraham (Hebrew) Father of a multitude; father of nations *Abarran, Avraham, Aberham, Abrahamo, Abrahan, Abrahim, Abram, Abrami, Ibrahim*

Abram (Hebrew) Form of Abraham, meaning "father of nations"

Adael (Hebrew) God witnesses *Adaele, Adayel, Adayele*

Adam (Hebrew) Of the earth *Ad, Adamo, Adams, Adan, Adao, Addam, Addams, Addem*

Adonis (Greek) In mythology, a handsome young man loved by Aphrodite *Addonia, Adohnes, Adonys*

Adrian (Latin) A man from Hadria *Adrien, Adrain, Adrean, Adreean, Adreyan, Adreeyan, Adriaan*

Adriel (Hebrew) From God's flock *Adriell, Adriele, Adryel, Adryell, Adryele*

Ahmad (Arabic) One who always thanks God; a name of Muhammed *Ahmed*

Aidan (Irish) A fiery young man *Aiden, Aedan, Aeden, Aidano, Aidyn, Ayden, Aydin, Aydan*

Ainsworth (English) From Ann's estate *Answorth, Annsworth, Ainsworthe, Answorthe, Annsworthe*

Ajax (Greek) In mythology, a hero of the Trojan war *Aias, Aiastes, Ajaxx, Ajaxe*

Alan (German / Gaelic) One who is precious / resembling a little rock *Alain, Alann, Allan, Alson, Allin, Allen, Allyn*

Albert (German) One who is noble and bright *Alberto, Albertus, Alburt, Albirt, Aubert, Albyrt, Albertos, Albertino*

Alden (English) An old friend
Aldan, Aldin, Aldyn, Aldon, Aldun

Aldo (German) Old or wise
one; elder *Aldous, Aldis, Aldus,*
Alldo, Aldys

Alejandro (Spanish) Form of
Alexander, meaning "a helper
and defender of mankind"
Alejandrino, Alejo

Alex (English) Form of
Alexander, meaning "a helper
and defender of mankind"
Aleks, Alecks, Alecs, Allex, Alleks,
Allecks, Alexis

Alexander (Greek) A helper
and defender of mankind
Alex, Alec, Alejandro, Alaxander,
Aleksandar, Aleksander,
Aleksandr, Alessandro,
Alexzander, Zander

Alfonso (Italian) Prepared
for battle; eager and ready
Alphonso, Alphonse, Affonso,
Alfons, Alfonse, Alfonsin,
Alfonsino, Alfonz, Alfonzo

Ali (Arabic) The great one;
one who is exalted *Alie, Aly,*
Aley, Alee

Alijah (American) Form of
Elijah, meaning "Jehovah is
my god"

Alton (English) From the old
town *Aldon, Aldun, Altun, Alten,*
Allton, Alltun, Allten

Amari (African) Having great
strength; a builder *Amare,*
Amarie, Amaree, Amarea, Amary,
Amarey

Amos (Hebrew) To carry; hardworking *Amoss, Aymoss, Aymos*

Andre (French) Form of Andrew, meaning "manly, a warrior" *Andreas, Andrei, Andrej, Andres, Andrey*

Andrew (Greek) One who is manly; a warrior *Andy, Aindrea, Andreas, Andie, Andonia, Andor, Andresj, Anderson, Anders*

Angel (Greek) A messenger of God *Andjelko, Ange, Angelino, Angell, Angelmo, Angelo, Angie, Angy*

Angus (Scottish) One force; one strength; one choice *Aengus, Anngus, Aonghus*

Anthony (Latin) A flourishing man; of an ancient Roman family *Antal, Antony, Anthoney, Anntoin, Antin, Anton, Antone, Antonello, Antonio*

Antoine (French) Form of Anthony, meaning "a flourishing man; of an ancient Roman family" *Antione, Antjuan, Antuan, Antuwain, Antuwaine, Antuwayne, Antuwon, Antwahn*

Antonio (Italian) Form of Anthony, meaning "a flourishing man, from an ancient Roman family" *Antonin, Antonino, Antonius, Antonyo*

Archer (Latin) A skilled bowman

Ari (Hebrew) Resembling a lion or an eagle *Aree, Arie, Aristide, Aristides, Arri, Ary, Arye, Arrie*

Ariel (Hebrew) A lion of God *Arielle, Ariele, Ariell, Arriel, Ahriel, Airial, Arieal, Arial*

Arnold (German) The eagle ruler *Arnaldo, Arnaud, Arnauld, Arnault, Arnd, Arndt, Arnel, Arnell*

Arthur (Celtic) As strong as a bear; a hero *Aart, Arrt, Art, Artair, Arte, Arther, Arthor, Arthuro*

Asa (Hebrew) One who heals others *Asah*

Ash (English) From the ash tree *Ashe*

Asher (Hebrew) Filled with happiness *Ashar, Ashor, Ashir, Ashyr, Ashur*

Asher

We named our son Asher because my grandmother's maiden name is Assh and we wanted to honor that branch of our family, many of whom are quite elderly. Also, my husband's name is Dan (not Daniel), which is one of the twelve tribes of Israel, and we liked the fact that Asher is one of the twelve tribes too. —Jackie, Montreal

Atticus (Latin) A man from Athens *Attikus, Attickus, Aticus, Atickus, Atikus*

Aubrey (English) One who rules with elf wisdom *Aubary, Aube, Aubery, Aubry, Aubury, Aubrian, Aubrien, Aubrion*

Auburn (Latin) Having a reddish-brown color *Aubirn, Auburne, Aubyrn, Abern, Abirn, Aburn, Abyrn, Aubern*

August (Irish) One who is venerable; majestic *Austin, Augustine, Agoston, Aguistin, Agustin, Augustin, Augustyn, Avgustin, Augusteen, Agosteen*

Austin (English) Form of August, meaning "one who is venerable; majestic" *Austen, Austyn, Austan, Auston, Austun*

Avery (English) One who is a wise ruler; of the nobility *Avrie, Averey, Averie, Averi, Averee*

Axel (German / Latin / Hebrew) Source of life; small oak / ax / peace *Aksel, Ax, Axe, Axell, Axil, Axill, Axl*

Ayden (Irish) Form of Aiden, meaning "a fiery young man"

B

Bain (Irish) A fair-haired man *Baine, Bayn, Bayne, Baen, Baene, Bane, Baines, Baynes*

Barak (Hebrew) Of the lightning flash *Barrak, Barac, Barrac, Barack, Barrack*

Barden (English) From the barley valley; from the boar's valley *Bardon, Bardun, Bardin, Bardyn, Bardan, Bardene*

Baron (English) A title of nobility *Barron*

Barry (Gaelic) A fair-haired man *Barrey, Barri, Barrie, Barree, Barrea, Barrington, Barryngton, Barringtun*

Bartholomew (Aramaic) The son of the farmer *Bart, Bartel, Barth, Barthelemy, Bartho, Barthold, Bartholoma, Bartholomaus, Bartlett, Bartol*

Bartlett (French) Form of Bartholomew, meaning "the son of the farmer" *Bartlet, Bartlitt, Bartlit, Bartlytt, Bartlyt*

Beau (French) A handsome man, an admirer *Bo*

Beckett (English) From the small stream; from the brook *Becket*

Ben (English) Form of Benjamin, meaning "son of the south; son of the right hand" *Benn, Benni, Bennie, Bennee, Benney, Benny, Bennea, Benno*

Benjamin (Hebrew) Son of the south; son of the right hand *Ben, Benejamen, Beniamino, Benjaman, Benjamen, Benjamino, Benjamon, Benjiman, Benjimen*

Bennett (English) Form of Benedict, meaning "one who is blessed" *Benett, Bennet, Benet*

Bentley (English) From the meadow of bent grass *Bently, Bentleigh, Bentlee, Bentlie*

Bernard (German) As strong and brave as a bear *Barnard, Barnardo, Barnhard, Barnhardo, Bearnard, Bernardo, Bernarr, Bernd*

Bennett

My husband Brent and I ran off and eloped in Florida. I jokingly told Brent's cousin, Jason Isaac, that I would name our first son after him if he came to our wedding. He and some other friends surprised us by attending! Our son is named Bennett Isaac. Bennett is my maiden name.
—Cynthia, MI

Blaine (Scottish / Irish) A saint's servant / a thin man *Blayne, Blane, Blain, Blayn, Blaen, Blaene, Blainy, Blainey*

Blaise (Latin / American) One with a lisp or a stutter / a fiery man *Blaze, Blaize, Blaiz, Blayze, Blayz, Blaez, Blaeze*

Blake (English) A dark, handsome man *Blayk, Blayke, Blaik, Blaike, Blaek, Blaeke*

Bob (English) Form of Robert, meaning "one who is bright with fame" *Bobbi, Bobbie, Bobby, Bobbey, Bobbee, Bobbea*

Bodhi (Buddhist) To become aware *Bode, Bodie*

Booker (English) One who binds books; a scribe *Bookar, Bookir, Bookyr, Bookur, Bookor*

Bosley (English) From the meadow near the forest *Bosly, Boslee, Boslea, Bosleah, Bosleigh, Bosli, Boslie, Bozley*

Boyd (Celtic) A blond-haired man *Boyde, Boid, Boide, Boyden, Boydan, Boydin, Boydyn, Boydon*

Braden (Gaelic / English) Resembling salmon / from the wide valley *Bradan, Bradon, Bradin, Bradyn, Braeden, Brayden*

Bradford (English) From the wide ford *Bradforde, Bradferd, Bradferde*

Bradley (English) From the wide meadow *Bradly, Bradlea, Bradleah, Bradlee, Bradleigh, Bradli*

Brady (Irish) The son of a large-chested man *Bradey, Bradee, Bradea, Bradi, Bradie, Braidy, Braidey, Braidee*

Brandon (English) From the broom or gorse hill *Brandun, Brandin, Brandyn, Brandan, Branden, Brannon, Brannun, Brannen*

Brant (English) Steep, tall

Brantley (English) Form of Brant, meaning "steep, tall" *Brantly*

Brendan (Irish) Born to royalty; a prince *Brendano, Brenden, Brendin, Brendon, Brendyn, Brendun*

Brennan (Gaelic) A sorrowful man; a teardrop *Brenan, Brenn, Brennen, Brennin, Brennon, Brenin, Brennun, Brennyn*

Brent (English) From the hill *Brendt, Brennt, Brentan, Brenten, Brentin, Brenton, Brentun, Brentyn*

Brett (Latin) A man from Britain or Brittany *Bret, Breton, Brette, Bretton, Brit, Briton, Britt, Brittain*

Brian (Gaelic / Celtic) Of noble birth / having great strength *Briano, Briant, Brien, Brion, Bryan, Bryant, Bryen, Bryent*

Briar (English) Resembling a thorny plant *Brier, Bryar, Bryer*

Brock (English) Resembling a badger *Broc*

Broderick (English) From the wide ridge *Broderik, Broderic, Brodrick, Brodryk, Brodyrc, Brodrik, Broderyc, Brodrig*

Brody (Gaelic / Irish) From the ditch *Brodie, Brodey, Brodi, Brodee*

Brooks (English) From the running stream *Brookes*

Bruce (Scottish) A man from Brieuse; one who is well-born; from an influential family *Brouce, Brooce, Bruci, Brucie, Brucey, Brucy*

Bruno (German) A brown-haired man *Brunoh, Brunoe, Brunow, Brunowe, Bruin, Bruine, Brunon, Brunun*

Bryce (Scottish / Anglo-Saxon) One who is speckled / the son of a nobleman *Brice, Bricio, Brizio, Brycio*

Bryson (Welsh) The son of Brice *Brisen, Brysin, Brysun, Brysyn, Brycen*

Byron (English) One who lives near the cow sheds *Byrom, Beyren, Beyron, Biren, Biron, Buiron, Byram, Byran*

C

Cade (English / French) One who is round / of the cask *Caid, Caide, Cayd, Cayde, Caed, Caede*

Cadmus (Greek) A man from the east; in mythology, the man who founded Thebes *Cadmar, Cadmo, Cadmos, Cadmuss*

Caesar (Latin) An emperor *Caezar, Casar, Cezar, Chezare, Caesarius, Ceasar, Ceazer*

Cain (Hebrew) One who wields a spear; something acquired; in the Bible, Adam and Eve's first son who killed his brother Abel *Cayn, Caen, Cane, Caine, Cayne, Caene*

Cale (English) Form of Charles, meaning "one who is manly and strong" *Cail, Caile, Cayl, Cayle, Cael, Caele*

Caleb (Hebrew) Resembling a dog *Cayleb, Caileb, Caeleb, Calob, Cailob, Caylob, Caelob, Kaleb*

Callum (Gaelic) Resembling a dove *Calum*

Calvin (French) The little bald one *Cal, Calvyn, Calvon, Calven, Calvan, Calvun, Calvino*

Camden (Gaelic) From the winding valley *Camdene, Camdin, Camdyn, Camdan, Camdon, Camdun*

Cameron (Scottish) Having a crooked nose *Cameren, Cameran, Camerin, Cameryn, Camerun, Camron, Camren, Camran, Tameron*

Campbell (Scottish) Having a crooked mouth *Campbel, Cambell, Cambel, Camp, Campe, Cambeul, Cambeull, Campbeul*

Carl (German) Form of Karl, meaning "a free man" *Carel, Carlan, Carle, Carlens, Carlitis, Carlin, Carlo, Carlos*

Carlos (Spanish) Form of Karl, meaning "a free man" *Carolos, Carolo, Carlito*

Carlsen (Scandinavian) The son of Carl *Carlssen, Carlson, Carlsson, Carlsun, Carllsun, Carlsin, Carllsin, Carlsyn*

Carlton (English) From the free man's town *Carltun, Carltown, Carston, Carstun, Carstown, Carleton, Carletun, Carlten*

Carmichael (Scottish) A follower of Michael

Carson (Scottish) The son of a marsh dweller *Carsen, Carsun, Carsan, Carsin, Carsyn*

Carter (English) One who transports goods; one who drives a cart *Cartar, Cartir, Cartyr, Cartor, Cartur, Cartere, Cartier, Cartrell*

Cary (Celtic / Welsh / Gaelic) From the river / from the fort on the hill / having dark features *Carey, Cari, Carie, Caree, Carea, Carry, Carrey, Carri*

Cash (Latin) Money

Cason (Greek) A seer
Casen, Kaysen

Cassius (Latin) One who is
empty; hollow; vain *Cassios,
Cassio, Cach, Cache, Cashus,
Cashos, Cassian, Cassien*

Cato (Latin) One who is all-
knowing *Cayto, Caito, Caeto*

Cesar (Spanish) Form of
Caesar, meaning "emperor"
Cesare, Cesaro, Cesario

Chad (English) One who
is warlike *Chaddie, Chadd,
Chadric, Chadrick, Chadrik,
Chadryck, Chadryc, Chadryk*

Chadwick (English) From
Chad's dairy farm *Chadwik,
Chadwic, Chadwyck, Chadwyk,
Chadwyc*

Chance (English) Having
good fortune

Chandler (English) One
who makes candles *Chandlar,
Chandlor*

Channing (French / English)
An official of the church /
resembling a young wolf
Channyng, Canning, Cannyng

Charles (English / German)
One who is manly and strong
/ a free man *Charls, Chas,
Charli, Charlie, Charley, Charly,
Charlee, Charleigh, Cale, Chuck,
Chick*

Charlie

We chose to name our son Charlie after his grandfather. But it seemed just right since we have a beagle—just like Charlie Brown and his beagle, Snoopy. —Maggie, IL

Charlton (English) From the free man's town *Charleton, Charltun, Charletun, Charleston, Charlestun*

Chase (English) A huntsman *Chace, Chasen, Chayce, Chayse, Chaise, Chaice, Chaece, Chaese*

Chelsey (English) From the landing place for chalk *Chelsee, Chelseigh, Chelsea, Chelsi, Chelsie, Chelsy, Chelcey, Chelcy*

Chester (Latin) From the camp of the soldiers *Chet, Chess, Cheston, Chestar, Chestor, Chestur, Chestir, Chestyr*

Christian (Greek) A follower of Christ *Chrestien, Chretien, Chris, Christan, Christer, Christiano, Cristian*

Christian

I wanted to name my son Christopher but my husband didn't want a name that common. We compromised on Christian so that he could shorten it to Chris if he didn't like his full name. To be honest, it is still growing on me. I am not sure I like that his name is a common noun and is regularly mistyped as "Christina." —Laura, WA

Christopher (Greek) One who bears Christ inside *Chris, Kit, Christof, Christofer, Christoffer, Christoforo, Christoforus, Christoph, Christophe, Cristopher, Cristofer*

Chuck (English) Form of Charles, meaning "one who is manly and strong / a free man" *Chucke, Chucki, Chuckie, Chucky, Chuckey, Chuckee, Chuckea*

Clancy (Celtic) Son of the red-haired warrior *Clancey, Clanci, Clancie, Clancee, Clancea, Clansey, Clansy, Clansi*

Clark (English) A cleric; a clerk *Clarke, Clerk, Clerke, Clerc*

Claude (English) One who is lame *Claud, Claudan, Claudell, Claidianus, Claudicio, Claudien, Claudino, Claudio*

Clay (English) Of the earth's clay

Clayton (English) From the town settled on clay *Claytun, Clayten, Claytin, Claytyn, Claytan, Cleyton, Cleytun, Cleytan*

Clifford (English) From the ford near the cliff *Cliff, Clyfford, Cliford, Clyford*

Clinton (English) From the town on the hill *Clynton, Clintun, Clyntun, Clint, Clynt, Clinte, Clynte*

Clive (English) One who lives near the cliff *Clyve, Cleve*

Cody (Irish / English) One who is helpful; a wealthy man / acting as a cushion *Codi, Codie, Codey, Codee, Codeah, Codea, Codier, Codyr*

Colby (English) From the coal town *Colbey, Colbi, Colbie, Colbee, Collby, Coalby, Colbea, Colbeah*

Cole (English) Having dark features; having coal-black hair *Coley, Coli, Coly, Colie, Colee, Coleigh, Colea, Colson*

Colin (Scottish) A young man; a form of Nicholas, meaning "of the victorious people" *Cailean, Colan, Colyn, Colon, Colen, Collin, Collan*

Colton (English) From the coal town *Colten, Coltun, Coltan, Coltin, Coltyn, Coltrain*

Conan (English / Gaelic) Resembling a wolf / one who is high and mighty *Conant*

Connery (Scottish) A daring man *Connary, Connerie, Conneri, Connerey, Connarie, Connari, Connarey, Conary*

Connor (Gaelic) A wolf lover *Conor, Conner, Coner, Connar, Conar, Connur, Conur, Connir, Conir*

Conroy (Irish) A wise adviser *Conroye, Conroi*

Constantine (Latin) One who is steadfast; firm *Dinos*

Cooper (English) One who makes barrels *Coop, Coopar, Coopir, Coopyr, Coopor, Coopur, Coopersmith, Cupere*

Corey (Irish) From the hollow; of the churning waters *Cory, Cori, Corie, Coree, Corea, Correy, Corry, Corri*

Cortez (Spanish) A courteous man *Cortes*

Covington (English) From the town near the cave *Covyngton, Covingtun, Covyngtun*

Craig (Gaelic) From the rocks; from the crag *Crayg, Craeg, Craige, Crayge, Craege, Crage, Crag*

Crawford (English) From the crow's ford *Crawforde, Crawferd, Crawferde, Crawfurd, Crawfurde*

Cruz (Spanish) Of the cross

Cullen (Gaelic) A good-looking young man *Cullin, Cullyn, Cullan, Cullon, Cullun*

D

Dacey (Gaelic / Latin) A man from the south / a man from Dacia *Dacy, Dacee, Dacea, Daci, Dacie, Daicey, Daicy*

Dakota (Native American) A friend to all *Daccota, Dakoda, Dakodah, Dakotah, Dakoeta, Dekota, Dekohta, Dekowta*

Dallas (Scottish) From the dales *Dalles, Dallis, Dallys, Dallos*

Dalton (English) From the town in the valley *Daltun, Dalten, Daltan, Daltin, Daltyn, Daleten, Dalte, Daulten*

Damian (Greek) One who tames or subdues others *Daemon, Daimen, Daimon, Daman, Damen, Dameon, Damiano, Damianos, Damon*

Dane (English) A man from Denmark *Dain, Daine, Dayn, Dayne*

Daniel (Hebrew) God is my judge *Dan, Danal, Daneal, Danek, Danell, Danial, Daniele, Danil, Danilo*

Dante (Latin) An enduring man; everlasting *Dantae, Dantay, Dantel, Daunte, Dontae, Dontay, Donte, Dontae*

Darion (Greek) A gift *Darian, Darien, Dariun, Darrion, Darrian, Darrien, Daryon, Daryan*

Darius (Greek) A kingly man; one who is wealthy *Darias, Dariess, Dario, Darious, Darrius, Derrius, Derrious, Derrias*

Darnell (English) From the hidden place *Darnall, Darneil, Darnel, Darnele, Darnelle*

Darren (Gaelic / English) A great man / a gift from God *Darran, Darrin, Darryn, Darron, Darrun, Daren, Darin, Daran*

Dash (American) A charming man

David (Hebrew) The beloved one *Dave, Davey, Davi, Davidde, Davide, Davie, Daviel, Davin, Daoud*

Davis (English) The son of David *Davies, Daviss, Davys, Davyss*

Dawson (English) The son of David *Dawsan, Dawsen, Dawsin, Dawsun*

Dax (French) From the French town Dax *Daxton*

Dayton (English) From the sunny town

Deacon (Greek) The dusty one; a servant *Deecon, Deakon, Deekon, Deacun, Deecun, Deakun, Deekun, Deacan*

Dean (English) From the valley; a church official *Deane, Deen, Deene, Dene, Deans, Deens, Deani, Deanie*

Decker (German / Hebrew) One who prays / a piercing man *Deker, Decer, Dekker, Deccer, Deck, Decke*

Declan (Irish) The name of a saint

Delaney (Irish / French) The dark challenger / from the elder-tree grove *Delany, Delanee, Delanea, Delani, Delanie, Delainey, Delainy, Delaini*

Dennis (French) A follower of Dionysus *Den, Denies, Denis, Dennes, Dennet, Denney, Dennie, Denys, Dennys*

Derek (English) The ruler of the tribe *Dereck, Deric, Derick, Derik, Deriq, Derk, Derreck, Derrek, Derrick*

Dexter (Latin) A right-handed man; one who is skillful *Dextor, Dextar, Dextur, Dextir, Dextyr, Dexton, Dextun, Dexten*

Diego (Spanish) Form of James, meaning "he who supplants" *Dyego, Dago*

Dietrich (German) The ruler of the tribe *Dedrick*

Digby (Norse) From the town near the ditch *Digbey, Digbee, Digbea, Digbi, Digbie*

Dillon (Gaelic) Resembling a lion; a faithful man *Dillun, Dillen, Dillan, Dillin, Dillyn, Dilon, Dilan, Dilin*

Dixon (English) The son of Dick *Dixen, Dixin, Dixyn, Dixan, Dixun*

Dominick

We decided to name our son Dominick after my husband's grandfather. We were unable to tell him before he unexpectedly passed away six weeks prior to my due date. We like to think that Papa knows and spends some time watching over our little boy. —Dawn, PA

Dominic (Latin) A lord *Demenico, Dom, Domenic, Domenico, Domenique, Domini, Dominick, Dominico*

Donald (Scottish) Ruler of the world *Don, Donold, Donuld, Doneld, Donild, Donyld*

Donovan (Irish) A brown-haired chief *Donavan, Donavon, Donevon, Donovyn*

Doran (Irish) A stranger; one who has been exiled *Doren, Dorin, Doryn*

Drake (English) Resembling a dragon *Drayce, Drago, Drakie*

Drew (Welsh) One who is wise *Drue, Dru*

Drummond (Scottish) One who lives on the ridge *Drummon, Drumond, Drumon, Drummund, Drumund, Drummun*

Duane (Gaelic) A dark or swarthy man *Dewain, Dewayne, Duante, Duayne, Duwain, Duwaine, Duwayne, Dwain*

Duke (English) A title of nobility; a leader *Dooke, Dook, Duki, Dukie, Dukey, Duky, Dukee, Dukea*

Duncan (Scottish) A dark warrior *Dunkan, Dunckan, Dunc, Dunk, Dunck*

Dustin (English / German) From the dusty area / a courageous warrior *Dustyn, Dusten, Dustan, Duston, Dustun, Dusty, Dustey, Dusti*

Dwight (Flemish) A white- or blond-haired man *Dwite, Dwhite, Dwyght, Dwighte*

Dylan (Welsh) Son of the sea *Dyllan, Dylon, Dyllon, Dylen, Dyllen, Dylun, Dyllun, Dylin*

E

Eagan (Irish) A fiery man
Eegan, Eagen, Eegen, Eagon,
Eegon, Eagun, Eegun

Eamon (Irish) Form of
Edmund, meaning "a wealthy
protector" *Eaman, Eamen,*
Eamin, Eamyn, Eamun, Eamonn,
Eames, Eemon

Ean (Gaelic) Form of John,
meaning "God is gracious"
Eion, Eyan, Eyon, Eian

Earl (English) A nobleman
Earle, Erle, Erl, Eorl

Easton (English) Eastern
place *Eastan, Easten, Eastyn*

Ed (English) Form of Edward,
meaning "a wealthy protector"
Edd, Eddi, Eddie, Eddy, Eddey,
Eddee, Eddea, Edi

Edgar (English) A powerful
and wealthy spearman *Eadger,*
Edgardo, Edghur, Edger

Edison (English) Son of
Edward *Eddison, Edisun,*
Eddisun, Edisen, Eddisen, Edisyn,
Eddisyn, Edyson

Edmund (English) A wealthy
protector *Ed, Eddie, Edmond,*
Eamon

Edward (English) A wealthy
protector *Ed, Eadward, Edik,*
Edouard, Eduard, Eduardo,
Edvard, Edvardas, Edwardo

Edwin (English) A wealthy friend *Edwinn, Edwinne, Edwine, Edwyn, Edwynn, Edwynne, Edwen, Edwenn*

Efrain (Spanish) Form of Ephraim, meaning "one who is fertile; productive" *Efraine, Efrayn, Efrayne, Efraen, Efraene, Efrane*

Eldorado (Spanish) The golden man

Eldred (English) An old, wise adviser *Eldrid, Eldryd, Eldrad, Eldrod, Edlrud, Ethelred*

Eli (Hebrew) One who has ascended; my God on High *Ely*

Elias (Hebrew) Form of Elijah, meaning "Jehovah is my god" *Eliyas*

Elijah (Hebrew) Jehovah is my God *Elija, Eliyahu, Eljah, Elja, Elyjah, Elyja, Elijuah, Elyjuah*

Elliott (English) Form of Elijah, meaning "Jehovah is my God" *Eliot, Eliott, Elliot, Elyot*

Elmo (English / Latin) A protector / an amiable man *Elmoe, Elmow, Elmowe*

Elroy (Irish / English) A red-haired young man / a king *Elroi, Elroye, Elric, Elryc, Elrik, Elryk, Elrick, Elryck*

Elton (English) From the old town *Ellton, Eltun, Elltun, Elten, Ellten, Eltin, Elltin, Eltyn*

Elvis (Scandinavian) One who is wise *Elviss, Elvys, Elvyss*

Emil (Latin) One who is eager; an industrious man *Emelen, Emelio, Emile, Emilian, Emiliano, Emilianus, Emilio, Emilion*

Emiliano (Spanish) Form of Emil, meaning "one who is eager"

Emmanuel (Hebrew) God is with us *Manuel, Manny, Em, Eman, Emmannuel*

Emmett (German) A universal man *Emmet, Emmit, Emmitt, Emmot*

Emrys (Welsh) An immortal man

Enrique (Spanish) The ruler of the estate *Enrico, Enriko, Enricko, Enriquez, Enrikay, Enreekay, Enrik, Enric*

Enzo (Italian) The ruler of the estate *Enzio, Enzeo, Enziyo, Enzeyo*

Ephraim (Hebrew) One who is fertile; productive *Eff, Efraim, Efram, Efrem, Efrain*

Eric (Scandinavian) Ever the ruler *Erek, Erich, Erick, Erik, Eriq, Erix, Errick, Eryk*

Ernest (English) One who is sincere and determined; serious *Earnest, Ernesto, Ernestus, Ernst, Erno, Ernie, Erni, Erney*

Esperanze (Spanish) Filled with hope *Esperance, Esperence, Esperenze, Esperanzo, Esperenzo*

Esteban (Spanish) One who is crowned in victory *Estebon, Estevan, Estevon, Estefan, Estefon, Estebe, Estyban, Estyvan*

Ethan (Hebrew) One who is firm and steadfast *Ethen, Ethin, Ethyn, Ethon, Ethun, Eitan, Etan, Eithan*

Eugene (Greek) A well-born man *Eugean, Eugenie, Ugene, Efigenio, Gene, Owen*

Evan (Welsh) Form of John, meaning "God is gracious" *Evann, Evans, Even, Evin, Evon, Evyn, Evian, Evien*

Everett (English) Form of Everhard, meaning "as strong as a bear" *Evered, Everet*

Ezekiel (Hebrew) Strengthened by God *Esequiel, Ezechiel, Eziechiele, Eziequel, Ezequiel, Ezekial, Ezekyel, Esquevelle, Zeke*

F

Fawcett (American) An audacious man *Fawcet, Fawcette, Fawcete, Fawce, Fawci, Fawcie, Fawcy, Fawcey*

Feivel (Hebrew) The brilliant one *Feival, Feivol, Feivil, Feivyl, Feivul, Feiwel, Feiwal, Feiwol*

Felipe (Spanish) Form of Phillip, meaning "one who loves horses" *Felippe, Filip, Filippo, Fillip, Flip, Fulop, Fullop, Fulip*

Felix (Latin) One who is happy and prosperous

Ferdinand (German) A courageous voyager *Ferdie, Ferdinando, Fernando*

Fergus (Gaelic) The first and supreme choice *Fearghas, Fearghus, Feargus, Fergie, Ferguson, Fergusson, Furgus, Fergy*

Finch (English) Resembling the small bird *Fynch, Finche, Fynche, Finchi, Finchie, Finchy, Finchey, Finchee*

Fineas (Egyptian) A dark-skinned man *Fyneas, Finius, Fynius*

Finian (Irish) A handsome man; fair *Finan, Finnian, Fionan, Finien, Finnien, Finghin, Finneen, Fineen*

Finn (Gaelic) A fair-haired
man *Fin, Fynn, Fyn, Fingal,
Fingall*

Finnegan (Irish) A fair-haired
man *Finegan, Finnegen, Finegen,
Finnigan, Finigan*

Fisher (English) A fisherman
Fischer, Fysher

Fitzgerald (English) The son
of Gerald *Fytzgerald*

Fletcher (English) One who
makes arrows *Fletch, Fletche,
Flecher*

Flynn (Irish) One who has a
ruddy complexion *Flyn, Flinn,
Flin, Flen, Flenn, Floinn*

Foley (English) A creative
man *Foly, Folee, Foli, Folie*

Frank (Latin) Form of Francis,
meaning "a man from France;
one who is free" *Franco, Frankie*

Fred (German) Form of
Frederick, meaning "a peace-
ful ruler" *Freddi, Freddie, Freddy,
Freddey, Freddee, Freddea,
Freddis, Fredis*

Frederick (German) A peace-
ful ruler *Fred, Fredrick, Federico,
Federigo, Fredek, Frederic,
Frederich, Frederico, Frederik,
Fredric*

Fullerton (English) From
Fuller's town *Fullertun, Fullertin,
Fullertyn, Fullertan, Fullerten*

G

Gabriel (Hebrew) A hero of God *Gabrian, Gabriele, Gabrielli, Gabriello, Gaby, Gab, Gabbi, Gabbie*

Gage (French) Of the pledge *Gaige, Gaege, Gauge*

Gale (Irish / English) A foreigner / one who is cheerful *Gail, Gaill, Gaille, Gaile, Gayl, Gayle, Gaylle, Gayll*

Galen (Greek) A healer; one who is calm *Gaelan, Gaillen, Galan, Galin, Galyn, Gaylen, Gaylin, Gaylinn*

Gallagher (Gaelic) An eager helper *Gallaghor, Gallaghar, Gallaghur, Gallaghir, Gallaghyr, Gallager, Gallagar, Gallagor*

Garcia (Spanish) One who is brave in battle *Garce, Garcy, Garcey, Garci, Garcie, Garcee, Garcea*

Garrett (English) Form of Gerard, meaning "one who is mighty with a spear" *Garett, Garret, Garretson, Garritt, Garrot, Garrott, Gerrit, Gerritt*

Garrison (French) Prepared *Garris, Garrish, Garry, Gary*

Garth (Scandinavian) The keeper of the garden *Garthe, Gart, Garte*

Garvin (English) A friend with a spear *Garvyn, Garven, Garvan, Garvon, Garvun*

Gary (English) One who wields a spear *Garey, Gari, Garie, Garea, Garee, Garry, Garrey, Garree*

Gaston (French) A man from Gascony *Gastun, Gastan, Gasten, Gascon, Gascone, Gasconey, Gasconi, Gasconie*

Gavin (Welsh) A little white falcon *Gavan, Gaven, Gavino, Gavyn, Gavynn, Gavon, Gavun, Gavyno*

Gene (English) Form of Eugene, meaning "a well-born man" *Genio, Geno, Geneo, Gino, Ginio, Gineo*

Geoffrey (English) Form of Jeffrey, meaning "a man of peace" *Geffrey, Geoff, Geoffery, Geoffroy, Geoffry, Geofrey, Geofferi, Geofferie*

George (Greek) One who works the earth; a farmer *Georas, Geordi, Geordie, Georg, Georges, Georgi, Georgie, Georgio, Yegor, Jurgen, Joren*

Gerald (German) One who rules with the spear *Jerald, Garald, Garold, Gearalt, Geralde, Geraldo, Geraud, Gere, Gerek*

Gerard (French) One who is mighty with a spear *Gerord, Gerrard, Gared, Garrett*

Germain (French / Latin) A man from Germany / one who is brotherly *Germaine, German, Germane, Germanicus, Germano, Germanus, Germayn, Germayne*

Gerry (German) Short form of names beginning with Ger–, such as Gerald or Gerard *Gerrey, Gerri, Gerrie, Gerrea, Gerree*

Gideon (Hebrew) A mighty warrior; one who fells trees *Gideone, Gidi, Gidon, Gidion, Gid, Gidie, Gidy, Gidey*

Gilbert (French / English) Of the bright promise / one who is trustworthy *Gib, Gibb, Gil, Gilberto, Gilburt, Giselbert, Giselberto, Giselbertus*

Giles (Greek) Resembling a young goat *Gyles, Gile, Gil, Gilles, Gillis, Gilliss, Gyle, Gyl*

Gill (Gaelic) A servant *Gyll, Gilly, Gilley, Gillee, Gillea, Gilli, Gillie, Ghill*

Giovanni (Italian) Form of John, meaning "God is gracious" *Geovani, Geovanney, Geovanni, Geovanny, Geovany, Giannino, Giovan, Giovani, Yovanny*

Giuseppe (Italian) Form of Joseph, meaning "God will add" *Giuseppi, Giuseppie, Giuseppy, Giuseppee, Giuseppea, Giuseppey, Guiseppe, Guiseppi*

Glen (Gaelic) From the secluded, narrow valley *Glenn, Glennard, Glennie, Glennon, Glenny, Glin, Glinn, Glyn*

Godfrey (German) God is peace *Giotto, Godefroi, Godfry, Godofredo, Goffredo, Gottfrid, Gottfried, Godfried*

Gordon (Gaelic) From the great hill; a hero *Gorden, Gordin, Gordyn, Gordun, Gordan, Gordi, Gordie, Gordee*

Grady (Gaelic) One who is famous; noble *Gradey, Gradee, Gradea, Gradi, Gradie, Graidy, Graidey, Graidee*

Grant

Our quest to come up with another one-syllable name for our son (his big sisters are Kate and Brooke) eventually led to an Elite Eight list of names on the delivery-room ink board. We eliminated the names of people we knew too well—Mitch, Josh, Scott, and Ross—and a couple others—Heath, Drake—before picking Grant. —Cam, CA

Graham (English) From the graveled area; from the gray home *Graem*

Granger (English) A farmer *Grainger, Graynger, Graenger, Grange, Graynge, Graenge, Grainge, Grangere*

Grant (English) A tall man; a great man *Grante, Graent*

Gray (English) A gray-haired man *Graye, Grai, Grae, Greye, Grey, Graylon, Graylen, Graylin*

Grayson (English) The son of a gray-haired man *Graysen, Graysun, Graysin, Greyson, Graysan, Graison, Graisun, Graisen*

Gregory (Greek) One who is vigilant; watchful *Greg, Greggory, Greggy, Gregori, Gregorie, Gregry, Grigori*

Griffin (Latin) Having a hooked nose *Griff, Griffen, Griffon, Gryffen, Gryffin, Gryphen*

Griffith (Welsh) A mighty chief *Griffyth, Gryffith, Gryffyth*

Gunner (Scandinavian) A bold warrior *Gunnar, Gunnor, Gunnur, Gunnir, Gunnyr*

Gus (German) A respected man; one who is exalted *Guss*

Gustav (Scandinavian) Of the staff of the gods *Gus, Gustave, Gussie, Gustaf, Gustof, Tavin*

H

Hadden (English) From the heather-covered hill *Haddan, Haddon, Haddin, Haddyn, Haddun*

Hagen (Gaelic) One who is youthful *Haggen, Hagan, Haggan, Hagin, Haggin, Hagyn, Haggyn, Hagon*

Hal (English) A form of Henry, meaning "the ruler of the house"; a form of Harold, meaning "the ruler of an army"

Halley (English) From the hall near the meadow *Hally, Halli, Hallie, Halleigh, Hallee, Halleah, Hallea*

Hamilton (English) From the flat-topped hill *Hamylton, Hamiltun, Hamyltun, Hamilten, Hamylten, Hamelton, Hameltun, Hamelten*

Hank (English) Form of Henry, meaning "the ruler of the house" *Hanke, Hanks, Hanki, Hankie, Hankee, Hankea, Hanky, Hankey*

Harim (Arabic) A superior man *Hareem, Haream, Hariem, Hareim, Harym*

Harold (Scandinavian) The ruler of an army *Hal, Harald, Hareld, Harry, Darold*

Harper (English) One who plays or makes harps *Harpur, Harpar, Harpir, Harpyr, Harpor, Hearpere*

Harrington (English) From Harry's town; from the herring town *Harringtun, Harryngton, Harryngtun, Harington, Haringtun, Haryngton, Haryntun*

Harrison (English) The son of Harry *Harrisson, Harris, Harriss, Harryson*

Harvey (English / French) One who is ready for battle / a strong man *Harvy, Harvi, Harvie, Harvee, Harvea, Harv, Harve, Hervey*

Hawkins (English) Resembling a small hawk *Haukins, Hawkyns, Haukyn*

Hawthorne (English) From the hawthorn tree *Hawthorn*

Hayden (English) From the hedged valley *Haydan, Haydon, Haydun, Haydin, Haydyn, Haden, Hadan, Hadon*

Haye (Scottish) From the stockade *Hay, Hae, Hai*

Heath (English) From the untended land of flowering shrubs *Heathe, Heeth, Heethe*

Hector (Greek) One who is steadfast; in mythology, the prince of Troy *Hecter, Hekter, Heckter*

Henderson (Scottish) The son of Henry *Hendrie, Hendries, Hendron, Hendri, Hendry, Hendrey, Hendree, Hendrea*

Hendrick (English) Form of Henry, meaning "the ruler of the house" *Hendryck, Hendrik, Hendryk, Hendric, Hendryc, Hendrix*

Henry (German) The ruler of the house *Hal, Hank, Harry, Henny, Henree, Henri, Hanraoi, Hendrick, Henrik*

Herman (German) A soldier *Hermon, Hermen, Hermun, Hermin, Hermyn, Hermann, Hermie*

Holden (English) From a hollow in the valley *Holdan, Holdyn, Holdon*

Hollis (English) From the holly tree *Hollys, Holliss, Hollyss, Hollace, Hollice*

Howard (English) The guardian of the home *Howerd, Howord, Howurd, Howird, Howyrd, Howi, Howie, Howy*

Hunter

My father passed away while I was pregnant with our son. We had to find a name that started with an H. We felt Hunter was the perfect name. It's both modern yet fairly uncommon. We feel it signifies strength, independence, and masculinity.
—Wendy, Toronto

Hubert (German) Having a shining intellect *Hobart, Huberte, Huburt, Huburte, Hubirt, Hubirte, Hubyrt, Hubyrte, Hubie, Uberto*

Hunter (English) A great huntsman and provider *Huntar, Huntor, Huntur, Huntir, Huntyr, Hunte, Hunt, Hunting*

Hudson (English) The son of Hugh; from the river *Hudsun, Hudsen, Hudsan, Hudsin, Hudsyn*

I

Ian (Gaelic) Form of John, meaning "God is gracious" *Iain, Iaine, Iayn, Iayne, Iaen, Iaene, Iahn*

Ibrahim (Arabic) Form of Abraham, meaning "father of a multitude; father of nations" *Ibraheem, Ibraheim, Ibrahiem, Ibraheam, Ibrahym*

Ida (Anglo-Saxon) A king *Idah*

Ignatius (Latin) A fiery man; one who is ardent *Ignac, Ignace, Ignacio, Ignacius, Ignatious, Ignatz, Ignaz, Ignazio*

Igor (Scandinavian / Russian) A hero / Ing's soldier *Igoryok*

Ike (Hebrew) Form of Isaac, meaning "full of laughter" *Iki, Ikie, Iky, Ikey, Ikee, Ikea*

Iker (Basque) A visitor *Ikar, Ikir, Ikyr, Ikor, Ikur*

Ingram (Scandinavian) A raven of peace *Ingra, Ingrem, Ingrim, Ingrym, Ingrum, Ingrom, Ingraham, Ingrahame, Ingrams*

Iniko (African) Born during troubled times *Inicko, Inico, Inyko, Inycko, Inyco*

Irwin (English) A friend of the wild boar *Irwinn, Irwinne, Irwyn, Irwynne, Irwine, Irwen, Irwenn, Irwenne*

Isaac (Hebrew) Full of laughter *Ike, Isaack, Isaak, Isac, Isacco, Isak, Issac, Itzak*

Isaiah (Hebrew) God is my salvation *Isa, Isaia, Isais, Isia, Isiah, Issiah, Izaiah, Iziah*

Israel (Hebrew) God perseveres *Israeli, Israelie, Isreal, Izrael*

Ivan (Slavic) Form of John, meaning "God is gracious" *Ivann, Ivanhoe, Ivano, Iwan, Iban, Ibano, Ivanti, Ivantie*

Ives (Scandinavian) The archer's bow; of the yew wood *Ivair, Ivar, Iven, Iver, Ivo, Ivon, Ivor, Ivaire*

J

Jabari (African) A valiant man *Jabarie, Jabary, Jabarey, Jabaree, Jabarea*

Jace (Hebrew) God is my salvation *Jacen, Jacey, Jacian, Jacy, Jaice, Jayce, Jaece, Jase*

Jack (English) Form of John, meaning "God is gracious" *Jackie, Jackman, Jacko, Jacky, Jacq, Jacqin, Jak, Jaq*

Jackson (English) The son of Jack or John *Jacksen, Jacksun, Jacson, Jakson, Jaxen, Jaxon, Jaxun, Jaxson*

Jacob (Hebrew) He who supplants *Jake, James, Kuba, Iakovos, Yakiv, Yankel, Yaqub,* *Jaco, Jacobo, Jacobi, Jacoby, Jacobie, Jacobey, Jacobo*

Jaden (Hebrew / English) One who is thankful to God; God has heard / form of Jade, meaning "resembling the green gemstone" *Jaiden, Jadyn, Jaeden, Jaidyn, Jayden, Jaydon*

Jaime (Spanish) Form of James, meaning "he who supplants" *Jamie, Jaimee, Jaimey, Jaimi, Jaimie, Jaimy, Jamee*

Jake (English) Form of Jacob, meaning "he who supplants" *Jaik, Jaike, Jayk, Jayke, Jakey, Jaky*

Jalen (American) One who heals others; one who is tranquil *Jaylon, Jaelan, Jalon, Jaylan, Jaylen, Jalan, Jaylin*

Jamal (Arabic) A handsome man *Jamail, Jahmil, Jam, Jamaal, Jamy, Jamar*

James (Hebrew) Form of Jacob, meaning "he who supplants" *Jaimes, Jaymes, Jame, Jaym, Jaim, Jaem, Jaemes, Jamese, Jim, Jaime, Diego, Hagop, Hemi, Jakome*

Jameson (English) The son of James *Jaimison, Jamieson, Jaymeson, Jamison, Jaimeson, Jaymison, Jaemeson, Jaemison*

Jared (Hebrew) Of the descent; descending *Jarad, Jarod, Jarrad, Jarryd, Jarred, Jarrod, Jaryd, Jerod, Jerrad, Jered*

············· **James** ·············

We love traditional-sounding names, especially ones that run in our family. We named our son after my husband's grandfather, and still love it. When people asked about his name before he was born, I was surprised how consistently they said it was such a strong name. —Kristi, FL

Jason (Hebrew / Greek) God is my salvation / a healer; in mythology, the leader of the Argonauts *Jacen, Jaisen, Jaison, Jasen, Jasin, Jasun, Jayson, Jaysen*

Javier (Spanish) The owner of a new house *Javiero*

Jax (American) Form of Jackson, meaning "son of Jack or John"

Jay (Latin / Sanskrit) Resembling a jaybird / one who is victorious *Jae, Jai, Jaye, Jayron, Jayronn, Jey*

Jayce (American) Form of Jason, meaning "God is my salvation" *Jayse, Jace, Jase*

Jean (French) Form of John, meaning "God is gracious" *Jeanne, Jeane, Jene, Jeannot, Jeanot*

Jedidiah (Hebrew) One who is loved by God *Jedadiah, Jedediah, Jed, Jedd, Jedidiya, Jedidiyah, Jedadia, Jedadiya*

Jeffrey (English) A man of peace *Jeff, Geoffrey, Jeffery, Jeffree*

Jeremiah (Hebrew) One who is exalted by the Lord *Jeremia, Jeremias, Jeremija, Jeremiya, Jeremyah, Jeramiah, Jeramia, Jerram, Geremia*

Jeremy (Hebrew) Form of Jeremiah, meaning "one who is exalted by the Lord" *Jeramey, Jeramie, Jeramy, Jerami, Jereme, Jeromy*

Jerome (Greek) Of the sacred name *Jairome, Jeroen, Jeromo, Jeronimo, Jerrome, Jerom, Jerolyn, Jerolin, Hieronim*

Jesse (Hebrew) God exists; a gift from God; God sees all *Jess, Jessey, Jesiah, Jessie, Jessy, Jese, Jessi, Jessee*

Jesus (Hebrew) God is my salvation *Jesous, Jesues, Jesús, Xesus*

Jett (English) Resembling the jet-black lustrous gemstone *Jet, Jette*

Jim (English) Form of James, meaning "he who supplants" *Jimi, Jimmee, Jimmey, Jimmie, Jimmy, Jimmi, Jimbo*

Joab (Hebrew) The Lord is my father *Joabb, Yoav*

Joachim (Hebrew) One who is established by God; God will judge *Jachim, Jakim, Joacheim, Joaquim, Joaquin, Josquin, Joakim, Joakeen*

Joe (English) Form of Joseph, meaning "God will add" *Jo, Joemar, Jomar, Joey, Joie, Joee, Joeye*

Joel (Hebrew) Jehovah is God; God is willing

Joey (Hebrew) Form of Joseph *Joe, Joseph*

Johan (German) Form of John, meaning "God is gracious"

Jonah

Due to family reasons, we wanted our child to have a *J* name. We have a big family, so many of the *J* names have already been used. We decided on Jonah, as it is a traditional, but not commonly used, name. —Sarah, IA

John (Hebrew) God is gracious; in the Bible, one of the Apostles *Sean, Jack, Juan, Ian, Ean, Evan, Giovanni, Hanna, Hovannes, Iefan, Ivan, Jean, Xoan, Yochanan, Yohan, Johnn, Johnny, Jhonny*

Jonah (Hebrew) Resembling a dove; in the Bible, the man swallowed by a whale

Jonas (Greek) Form of Jonah, meaning "resembling a dove"

Jonathan (Hebrew) A gift of God *Johnathan, Johnathon, Jonathon, Jonatan, Jonaton, Jonathen, Johnathen, Jonaten, Yonatan*

Jordan (Hebrew) Of the downflowing river; in the Bible, the river where Jesus was baptized *Johrdan, Jordain, Jordaine, Jordane, Jordanke, Jordann, Jorden, Jordaen*

Jorge (Spanish) Form of George, meaning "one who works the earth; a farmer"

Joey

My husband has always told me that Italian tradition is that the first grandson should be named after the paternal grandfather. We wanted a more American name than my husband's father, Giuseppe, so we chose Joseph. We used my dad's name, Richard, for the middle name, so Joey is named after his grandfathers. —Dana, IL

Jose (Spanish) Form of Joseph, meaning "God will add" *José, Joseito, Joselito*

Joseph (Hebrew) God will add *Joe, Joey, Guiseppe, Yosyp, Jessop, Jessup, Joop, Joos, José, Jose, Josef, Joseito*

Joshua (Hebrew) God is salvation *Josh, Joshuah, Josua, Josue, Joushua, Jozua, Joshwa, Joshuwa*

Josiah (Hebrew) God will help *Josia, Josias, Joziah, Jozia, Jozias*

Juan (Spanish) Form of John, meaning "God is gracious" *Juanito, Juwan, Jwan*

Judah (Hebrew) One who praises God *Juda, Jude, Judas, Judsen, Judson, Judd, Jud*

Jude (Latin) Form of Judah, meaning "one who praises God"

Julian (Greek) The child of
Jove; one who is youthful
*Juliano, Julianus, Julien, Julyan,
Julio, Jolyon, Jullien, Julen*

Julius (Greek) One who is
youthful *Juleus, Yuliy*

Justice (English) One who
upholds moral rightness and
fairness *Justyce, Justiss, Justyss,
Justis, Justus, Justise*

Justin (Latin) One who is
just and upright *Joost, Justain,
Justan, Just, Juste, Justen,
Justino, Justo*

K

Kacey (Irish) A vigilant man; one who is alert *Kacy, Kacee, Kacea, Kaci, Kacie, Kasey, Kasy, Kasi*

Kaden (Arabic) A beloved companion *Kadan, Kadin, Kadon, Kaidan, Kaiden, Kaidon, Kaydan, Kayden*

Kai (Hawaiian / Welsh / Greek) Of the sea / the keeper of the keys / of the earth *Kye*

Kale (English) Form of Charles, meaning "one who is manly and strong / a free man"

Kaleb (Hebrew) Resembling an aggressive dog *Kaileb, Kaeleb, Kayleb, Kalob, Kailob, Kaelob*

Kamden (English) From the winding valley *Kamdun, Kamdon, Kamdan, Kamdin, Kamdyn*

Kane (Gaelic) The little warrior *Kayn, Kayne, Kaen, Kaene, Kahan, Kahane*

Karl (German) A free man *Carl, Karel, Karlan, Karle, Karlens, Karli, Karlin, Karlo, Karlos*

Karson (Scottish) Form of Carson, meaning "son of a marsh dweller" *Karsen*

Karter (English) Form of Carter, meaning "one who drives a cart"

Kason (Basque) Protected by a helmet *Kasin, Kasyn, Kasen, Kasun, Kasan*

Keanu (Hawaiian) Of the mountain breeze *Keanue, Kianu, Kianue, Keanoo, Kianoo, Keanou*

Keaton (English) From the town of hawks *Keatun, Keeton, Keetun, Keyton, Keytun*

Keegan (Gaelic) A small and fiery man *Kegan, Keigan, Keagan, Keagen, Keegen*

Keith (Scottish) Man from the forest *Keithe, Keath, Keathe, Kieth, Kiethe, Keyth, Keythe, Keithen*

Keaton

My fourth child was supposed to have been a girl, so we had no boy name picked out. The other kids all had six-letter, two-syllable names of cities, so we had to think hard to match! We all spent two days in the hospital trying to come up with a name, and Keaton was the only name that everyone liked. —Beth, IA

Kellen (Gaelic / German) One who is slender / from the swamp *Kellan, Kellon, Kellun, Kellin*

Kelley (Celtic / Gaelic) A warrior / one who defends *Kelly, Kelleigh, Kellee, Kellea, Kelleah, Kelli, Kellie*

Kendrick (English / Gaelic) A royal ruler / the champion *Kendric, Kendricks, Kendrik, Kendrix, Kendryck, Kenrick, Kenrik, Kenricks*

Kenley (English) From the king's meadow *Kenly, Kenlee, Kenleigh, Kenlea, Kenleah, Kenli, Kenlie*

Kenn (Welsh) Of the bright waters *Ken*

Kennedy (Gaelic) A helmeted chief *Kennedi, Kennedie, Kennedey, Kennedee, Kennedea, Kenadie, Kenadi, Kenady*

Kenneth (Irish) Born of the fire; an attractive man *Kennet, Kennett, Kennith, Kennit, Kennitt*

Kent (English) From the edge or border *Kentt, Kennt, Kentrell*

Kevin (Gaelic) A beloved and handsome man *Kevyn, Kevan, Keven, Keveon, Kevinn, Kevion, Kevis, Kevon*

Kieran (Gaelic) Having dark features; the little dark one *Keiran, Keiron, Kernan, Kieren, Kiernan, Kieron, Kierren, Kierrien, Kierron, Keeran, Keeron, Keernan, Keeren, Kearan, Kearen, Kearon, Kearnan*

Kincaid (Celtic) The leader during battle *Kincade, Kincayd, Kincayde, Kincaide, Kincaed, Kincaede, Kinkaid, Kinkaide*

King (English) The royal ruler *Kyng, Kingsley*

Kingston (English) From the king's town *Kingstun, Kinston, Kindon*

Kipp (English) From the small, pointed hill *Kip, Kipling, Kippling, Kypp, Kyp, Kiplyng, Kipplyng, Kippi*

Kirk (Norse) A man of the church *Kyrk, Kerk, Kirklin, Kirklyn*

Kit (English) Form of Christopher, meaning "one who bears Christ inside" *Kitt, Kyt, Kytt*

Knox (English) From the rounded hill

Kobe (African / Hungarian) Tortoise / form of Jacob, meaning "he who supplants" *Kobi, Koby*

Kody (English) One who is helpful *Kodey, Kodee, Kodea, Kodi, Kodie*

Kory (Irish) From the hollow; of the churning waters *Korey, Kori, Korie, Koree, Korea, Korry, Korrey, Korree*

Kramer (German) A shop-keeper *Kramar, Kramor, Kramir, Kramur, Kramyr, Kraymer, Kraimer, Kraemer*

Kristopher (Scandinavian) A follower of Christ *Khristopher, Kristof, Kristofer, Kristoff, Kristoffer, Kristofor, Kristophor, Krystof*

Kumar (Indian) A prince; a male child

Kyle (Gaelic) From the narrow channel *Kile, Kiley, Kye, Kylan, Kyrell, Kylen, Kily, Kili*

L

Lachlan (Gaelic) From the land of lakes *Lachlen, Lachlin, Lachlyn, Locklan, Locklen, Locklin, Locklyn, Loklan*

Lamar (German / French) From the renowned land / of the sea *Lamarr, Lamarre, Lemar, Lemarr*

Lance (English) Form of Lancelot, meaning "an attendant, a knight of the Round Table"

Landon (English) From the long hill *Landyn, Landan, Landen, Landin, Lando, Langdon, Langden, Langdan*

Lane (English) One who takes the narrow path *Laine, Lain, Laen, Laene, Layne, Layn*

Langston (English) From the tall man's town *Langsten, Langstun, Langstown, Langstin, Langstyn, Langstan, Langton, Langtun*

Larson (Scandinavian) The son of Lawrence *Larsan, Larsen, Larsun, Larsin, Larsyn*

Lasalle (French) From the hall *Lasall, Lasal, Lasale*

Laurian (English) One who lives near the laurel trees *Laurien, Lauriano, Laurieno, Lawrian, Lawrien, Lawriano, Lawrieno*

Lawler (Gaelic) A soft-spoken man; one who mutters *Lauler, Lawlor, Loller, Lawlar, Lollar, Loller, Laular, Laulor*

Lawrence (Latin) Man from Laurentum; crowned with laurel *Larance, Laranz, Larenz, Larrance, Larrence, Larrens, Larrey, Larry*

Leavitt (English) A baker *Leavit, Leavytt, Leavyt, Leavett, Leavet*

Lee (English) From the meadow *Leigh, Lea, Leah, Ley*

Leighton (English) From the town near the meadow *Leightun, Layton, Laytun, Leyton, Leytun*

Leland (English) From the meadow land

Lennon (English) Son of love *Lennan*

Lennox (Scottish) One who owns many elm trees *Lenox, Lenoxe, Lennix, Lenix, Lenixe*

Leo (Latin) Having the strength of a lion *Lio, Lyo, Leon*

Leon (Greek) Form of Leo, meaning "lion"

Leonard (German) Having the strength of a lion *Len, Lenard, Lenn, Lennard, Lennart, Lennerd, Leonardo*

Leroy (French) The king *Leroi, Leeroy, Leeroi, Learoy, Learoi*

Levi (Hebrew) We are united as one; in the Bible, one of Jacob's sons *Levie, Levin, Levyn, Levy, Levey, Levee*

Liam (Gaelic) Form of William, meaning "the determined protector"

Lincoln (English) From the village near the lake *Lincon, Lyncon, Linc, Lynk, Lync*

Logan (Gaelic) From the little hollow *Logann, Logen, Login, Logyn, Logenn, Loginn, Logynn*

Louis (German) A famous warrior *Lew, Lewes, Lewis, Lodewick, Lodovico, Lou, Louie, Lucho, Luis*

Lucas (English) A man from Lucania *Lukas, Loucas, Loukas, Luckas, Louckas, Lucus, Lukus, Ghoukas*

Lucian (Latin) Surrounded by light *Luciano, Lucianus, Lucien, Lucio, Lucjan, Lukianos, Lukyan, Luce*

Luis (Spanish) Form of Louis, meaning "a famous warrior" *Luiz*

Luke (Greek) A man from Lucania *Luc, Luken*

Luther (German) A soldier of the people *Louther, Luter, Luthero, Lutero, Louthero, Luthus, Luthas, Luthos*

Lynn (English) A man of the lake *Linn, Lyn, Lynne, Linne*

M

Mac (Gaelic) The son of
Mac (Macarthur, Mackinley,
etc.) *Mack, Mak, Macky, Macki,
Mackie, Mackee, Mackea*

Macallister (Gaelic) The son
of Alistair *MacAlister, McAlister,
McAllister, Macalister*

Maddox (Welsh) The son
of the benefactor *Madox,
Madocks, Maddocks, Maddux*

Maguire (Gaelic) The son
of the beige one *Magwire,
MacGuire, McGuire, MacGwire,
McGwire*

Malachi (Hebrew) A messen-
ger of God *Malachie, Malachy,
Malaki, Malakia, Malakie,
Malaquias, Malechy, Maleki*

Malcolm (Gaelic) Follower
of St. Columbus *Malcom,
Malcolum, Malkolm, Malkom,
Malkolum*

Marcel (French) The little
warrior *Marceau, Marcelin,
Marcellin, Marcellino, Marcell,
Marcello, Marcellus, Marcelo*

Marcus (Latin) Form of Mark,
meaning "dedicated to Mars,
the god of war" *Markus, Marcas,
Marco, Markos*

Mario (Latin) A manly man
*Marius, Marios, Mariano, Marion,
Mariun, Mareon*

Mark (Latin) Dedicated to Mars, the god of war *Marc, Markey, Marky, Marki, Markie, Markee, Markea, Markov*

Marshall (French / English) A caretaker of horses / a steward *Marchall, Marischal, Marischall, Marschal, Marshal, Marshell, Marshel, Marschall*

Martin (Latin) Dedicated to Mars, the god of war *Martyn, Mart, Martel, Martell, Marten, Martenn, Marti, Martie*

Marvin (Welsh) A friend of the sea *Marvinn, Marvinne, Marven, Marvenn, Marvenne, Marvyn, Marvynn, Marvynne, Mervin*

Mason (English) One who works with stone *Masun, Masen, Masan, Masin, Masyn, Masson, Massun, Massen, Maison*

······························ **Mason** ······························

We chose Mason because he was our first child and a boy, and because a mason is a "brick builder"; our Mason would be our foundation, the builder of our family. —Sheila, MO

···················· **Matthew** ····················

At a gathering two nights before my son was born, my family shot down every name I had picked out. When asked his choice, my husband said, "Matthew," a name he'd never mentioned before. I said, "Fine, no more discussion!" Matthew arrived two days later—five weeks early. He really is my "gift of the Lord." —Stephanie, MI

Matteo (Italian) Form of Matthew, meaning "a gift from God" *Mateo*

Matthew (Hebrew) A gift from God *Matt, Mathew, Matvey, Mateas, Mattix, Madteos, Matthias, Mat, Mateo, Matteo, Mateus*

Maurice (Latin) A dark-skinned man; Moorish *Maurell, Maureo, Mauricio, Maurids, Maurie, Maurin, Maurio, Maurise, Baurice*

Maverick (English) An independent man; a nonconformist *Maveric, Maverik, Mavrick, Mavric, Mavrik*

Max (English) Form of Maxwell, meaning "from Mack's spring"

Maximilian (Latin) The greatest *Max, Macks, Maxi, Maxie, Maxy, Maxey, Maxee, Maxea, Maximiliano*

Melvin (English) A friend who offers counsel *Melvinn, Melvinne, Melven, Melvenn, Melvenne, Melvyn, Melvynn, Melvynne, Belvin*

Memphis (American) From the city in Tennessee *Memfis, Memphys, Memfys, Memphus, Memfus*

Micah (Hebrew) Form of Michael, meaning "Who is like God?" *Mica, Mycah*

Michael (Hebrew) Who is like God? *Makai, Micael, Mical, Micha, Michaelangelo, Michail, Michal, Micheal, Miguel*

Mick (English) Form of Michael, meaning "Who is like God?" *Micke, Mickey, Micky, Micki, Mickie, Mickee, Mickea, Mickel*

Miguel (Portuguese / Spanish) Form of Michael, meaning "Who is like God?" *Migel, Myguel*

Miles (German / Latin) One who is merciful / a soldier *Myles, Miley, Mily, Mili, Milie, Milee*

Miller (English) One who works at the mill *Millar, Millor, Millur, Millir, Millyr, Myller, Millen, Millan*

Milo (German) Form of Miles, meaning "one who is merciful" *Mylo*

Mitchell (English) Form of Michael, meaning "Who is like God?" *Mitch, Mitchel, Mytch, Mitchum, Mytchill, Mitcham*

Mohammed (Arabic) One who is greatly praised; the name of the prophet and founder of Islam *Mahomet, Mohamad, Mohamed, Mohamet, Mohammad, Muhammad, Muhammed, Mehmet*

Monroe (Gaelic) From the mouth of the river Roe *Monro, Monrow, Monrowe, Munro, Munroe, Munrow, Munrowe*

Montgomery (French) From Gomeric's mountain *Monty, Montgomerey, Montgomeri, Montgomerie, Montgomeree, Montgomerea*

Mortimer (French) Of the still water; of the dead sea *Mortymer, Morty, Mortey, Morti, Mortie, Mortee, Mortea, Mort, Morte*

Moses (Hebrew) A savior; in the Bible, the leader of the Israelites; drawn from the water *Mioshe, Mioshye, Mohsen, Moke, Moise, Moises, Mose, Moshe*

Murphy (Gaelic) A warrior of the sea *Murphey, Murphee, Murphea, Murphi, Murphie, Murfey, Murfy, Murfee*

Murray (Gaelic) The lord of the sea *Murrey, Murry, Murri, Murrie, Murree, Murrea*

N

Nathan

We named our son Nathan Joseph, just because we liked it. We expected to only call him Nate, but we find ourselves using both. —Peter, IL

Nathan (Hebrew) Form of Nathaniel, meaning "a gift from God" *Nat, Natan, Nate, Nathen, Nathon, Nathin, Nathyn, Nathun, Lathan*

Nathaniel (Hebrew) A gift from God *Nathan, Natanael, Nataniel, Nathanael, Nathaneal, Nathanial, Nathanyal, Nathanyel, Nethanel*

Neil (Gaelic) The champion *Neal, Neale, Neall, Nealle, Nealon, Neel, Neilan, Neile*

Nelson (English) The son of Neil; the son of a champion *Nealson, Neilson, Neillson, Nelsen, Nilson, Nilsson, Nelli, Nellie*

Neville (French) From the new village *Nev, Nevil, Nevile, Nevill, Nevylle, Nevyl, Nevyle, Nevyll*

Nicholas (Greek) Of the victorious people *Nick, Nicanor, Niccolo, Nichol, Nicholai, Nicholaus, Nikolai, Nicholl, Nichols, Colin, Nicolas, Nico*

Nick (English) Form of Nicholas, meaning "of the victorious people" *Nik, Nicki, Nickie, Nickey, Nicky, Nickee, Nickea, Niki*

Noah (Hebrew) A peaceful wanderer *Noa*

Nolan (Gaelic) A famous and noble man; a champion of the people *Nolen, Nolin, Nolon, Nolun, Nolyn, Noland, Nolande*

North (English) A man from the north *Northe*

O

Oberon (German) A royal
bear; having the heart of a
bear *Oberron*

Olaf (Scandinavian) The
remaining of the ancestors
Olay, Ole, Olef, Olev, Oluf, Uolevi

Oliver (Latin) From the olive
tree *Oliviero, Olivero, Olivier,
Oliviero, Olivio, Ollie*

Omar (Arabic) A flourishing
man; one who is well-spoken
Omarr, Omer

Oren (Hebrew / Gaelic) From
the pine tree / a pale-skinned
man *Orenthiel, Orenthiell,
Orenthiele, Orenthielle,
Orenthiem, Orenthium, Orin*

Orion (Greek) A great hunter

Orson (Latin) Resembling a
bear; raised by a bear *Orsen,
Orsin, Orsini, Orsino, Orsis,
Orsonio, Orsinie, Orsiny*

Orville (French) From the
gold town *Orvell, Orvelle, Orvil,
Orvill, Orvele, Orvyll, Orvylle,
Orvyl*

Oscar (English / Gaelic) A
spear of the gods / a friend of
deer *Oskar, Osker, Oscer, Osckar,
Oscker, Oszkar, Oszcar*

Owen (Welsh / Gaelic) Form
of Eugene, meaning "a well-
born man" / a youthful man
*Owenn, Owenne, Owin, Owinn,
Owinne, Owyn, Owynn, Owynne*

Oz (Hebrew) Having great strength *Ozz, Ozzi, Ozzie, Ozzy, Ozzey, Ozzee, Ozzea, Ozi*

P

Palmer (English) A pilgrim bearing a palm branch *Pallmer, Palmar, Pallmar, Palmerston, Palmiro, Palmeero, Palmeer, Palmire*

Parker (English) The keeper of the park *Parkar, Parkes, Parkman, Park*

Pascal (Latin) Born during Easter *Pascale, Pascalle, Paschal, Paschalis, Pascoe, Pascual, Pascuale, Pasqual*

Patrick (Latin) A nobleman; patrician *Packey, Padric, Pat, Patrece, Patric, Patrice, Patreece, Patricio*

Patton (English) From the town of warriors *Paten, Patin, Paton, Patten, Pattin, Paddon, Padden, Paddin*

Paul (Latin) A small or humble man *Pauley, Paulie, Pauly, Paley, Paavo*

Paxton (English) From the peaceful town *Packston, Paxon, Paxten, Paxtun, Packstun, Packsten*

Pedro (Spanish) Form of Peter, meaning "as solid and strong as a rock" *Pedrio, Pepe, Petrolino, Piero, Pietro*

Percival (French) One who can pierce the vale *Purcival, Percy, Percey, Perci, Percie, Percee, Percea, Persy, Persey, Persi*

Peter (Greek) As solid and strong as a rock *Peder, Pekka, Per, Petar, Pete, Peterson, Petr, Petre, Pierce, Patch, Pedro*

Peyton (English) From the village of warriors *Payton, Peytun, Paytun, Peyten, Payten, Paiton, Paitun, Paiten*

Phillip (Greek) One who loves horses *Phil, Philip, Felipe, Filipp, Phillie, Philly*

Pierce (English) Form of Peter, meaning "as solid and strong as a rock" *Pearce, Pears, Pearson, Pearsson, Peerce, Peirce, Pierson, Piersson*

Prescott (English) From the priest's cottage *Prescot, Prestcot, Prestcott, Preostcot*

Preston (English) From the priest's town *Prestin, Prestyn, Prestan, Prestun, Presten, Pfeostun*

Q

Quaid (Irish) Form of Walter, meaning "the commander of the army" *Quaide, Quayd, Quayde, Quaed, Quaede*

Quentin (Latin) The fifth-born child *Quent, Quenten, Quenton, Quentun, Quentan, Quentyn, Quente, Qwentin*

Quillan (Gaelic) Resembling a cub *Quilan, Quillen, Quilen, Quillon, Quilon*

Quincy (English) The fifth-born child; from the fifth son's estate *Quincey, Quinci, Quincie, Quincee, Quinncy, Quinnci, Quyncy, Quyncey*

Quinlan (Gaelic) A strong and healthy man *Quindlan, Quinlen, Quindlen, Quinian, Quinlin, Quindlin, Quinlyn, Quindlyn*

Quinn (Gaelic) One who provides counsel; an intelligent man *Quin, Quinne, Qwinn, Quynn, Qwin, Quiyn, Quyn, Qwinne*

R

Rafe (Irish) A tough man
Raffe, Raff, Raf, Raif, Rayfe, Raife,
Raef, Raefe

Ralph (English) Wolf counsel *Ralf, Ralphe, Ralfe, Ralphi,*
Ralphie, Ralphee, Ralphea,
Ralphy, Raoul

Ramsey (English) From the raven island; from the island of wild garlic *Ramsay, Ramsie,*
Ramsi, Ramsee, Ramsy, Ramsea,
Ramzy, Ramzey

Randall (German) The wolf shield *Randy, Randal, Randale,*
Randel, Randell, Randl, Randle,
Randon, Rendall

Randolph (German) The wolf shield *Randy, Randolf, Ranolf,*
Ranolph, Ranulfo, Randulfo,
Randwulf, Ranwulf, Randwolf

Randy (English) Form of Randall or Randolph, meaning "the wolf shield" *Randey, Randi,*
Randie, Randee, Randea

Ravi (Hindi) From the sun *Ravie, Ravy, Ravey, Ravee, Ravea*

Ray (English) Form of Raymond, meaning "a wise protector" *Rae, Rai, Rayce,*
Rayder, Rayse, Raye, Rayford,
Raylen

Raymond (German) A wise protector *Ray, Raemond,*
Raemondo, Raimond, Raimondo,
Raimund, Raimundo, Rajmund,
Ramon

Reeve (English) A bailiff *Reve, Reave, Reeford, Reeves, Reaves, Reves, Reaford*

Regan (Gaelic) Born into royalty; the little ruler *Raegan, Ragan, Raygan, Reganne, Regann, Regane, Reghan, Reagan*

Reggie (Latin) Form of Reginald, meaning "the king's adviser" *Reggi, Reggy, Reggey, Reggea, Reggee, Reg*

Reginald (Latin) The king's adviser *Reggie, Reynold, Raghnall, Rainault, Rainhold, Raonull, Raynald, Rayniero, Regin, Reginaldo*

Reid (English) A red-haired man; one who lives near the reeds *Read, Reade, Reed, Reede, Reide, Raed*

Reilly (Gaelic) An outgoing man *Reilley, Reilli, Reillie, Reillee, Reilleigh, Reillea*

Remington (English) From the town of the raven's family *Remyngton, Remingtun, Remyngtun*

Reuben (Hebrew) Behold, a son! *Reuban, Reubin, Reuven, Rouvin, Rube, Ruben, Rubin, Rubino*

Rhett (Latin) A well-spoken man *Rett, Rhet*

Rhys (Welsh) Having great enthusiasm for life

Richard (English) A powerful ruler *Rick, Rich, Ricard, Ricardo, Riccardo, Richardo, Richart, Richerd, Rickard, Rickert*

Richmond (French / German) From the wealthy hill / a powerful protector *Richmonde, Richmund, Richmunde*

Rick (English) Form of Richard, meaning "a powerful ruler" *Ric, Ricci, Ricco, Rickie, Ricki, Ricky, Rico, Rik*

Riley (English) From the rye clearing *Ryly, Ryli, Rylie, Rylee, Ryleigh, Rylea, Ryleah*

Riordain (Irish) A bright man *Riordane, Riordayn, Riordaen, Reardain, Reardane, Reardayn, Reardaen*

River (American) From the river *Ryver, Rivers, Ryvers*

Robert (German) One who is bright with fame *Bob, Rupert, Riobard, Roban, Robers, Roberto, Robertson, Robartach*

Roderick (German) A famous ruler *Rod, Rodd, Roddi, Roddie, Roddy, Roddee, Roddea*

Rodney (German / English) From the famous one's island / from the island's clearing *Rodny, Rodni, Rodnie*

Roland (German) From the renowned land *Roeland, Rolando, Roldan, Roley, Rollan, Rolland, Rollie, Rollin*

Roman (Latin) A citizen of Rome *Romain, Romaine, Romeo*

Romeo (Italian) Traveler to Rome

Ronald (Norse) The king's adviser *Ranald, Renaldo, Ronal, Ronaldo, Rondale, Roneld, Ronell, Ronello*

Ronan (Gaelic) Resembling a little seal *Ronin*

Rory (Gaelic) A red-haired man *Rori, Rorey, Rorie, Rorea, Roree, Rorry, Rorrey, Rorri*

Roy (Gaelic / French) A red-haired man / a king *Roye, Roi, Royer, Ruy*

Rufus (Latin) A red-haired man *Ruffus, Rufous, Rufino*

Rupert (English) Form of Robert, meaning "one who is bright with fame" *Ruprecht*

Russell (French) A little red-haired boy *Russel, Roussell, Russ, Rusel, Rusell*

Ryan (Gaelic) The little ruler; little king *Rian, Rien, Rion, Ryen, Ryon, Ryun, Rhyan, Rhyen*

··························· **Ryan** ···························

When I was expecting, my husband and I couldn't decide on a name. He liked traditional names, and I wanted a more trendy one. When we came across Ryan, it was the perfect compromise—not too traditional and not too trendy. His middle name, Richard, honors my father, who passed away before my son was born. —Michelle, IN

Ryder (English) An accomplished horseman *Rider, Ridder, Ryden, Rydell, Rydder*

Ryker (Danish) Form of Richard, meaning "a powerful ruler" *Riker*

S

Salim (Arabic) One who is peaceful *Saleem, Salem, Selim*

Salvador (Spanish) A savior *Sal, Sally, Salvadore, Xalvador*

Samson (Hebrew) As bright as the sun; in the Bible, a man with extraordinary strength *Sampson, Sansom, Sanson, Sansone*

Samuel (Hebrew) God has heard *Sam, Sammie, Sammy, Samuele, Samuello, Samwell, Samuelo, Sammey*

Sanford (English) From the sandy crossing *Sandford, Sanforde, Sandforde, Sanfurd, Sanfurde, Sandfurd, Sandfurde*

Santiago (Spanish) Refers to St. James

·············· **Sam** ··············

We named our son Samuel Edward. We always loved the name Sam, and Edward is a tribute to Sam's grandfather. We're so happy we chose that name. He's really grown into it! —Elaine, IL

Sawyer (English) One who works with wood *Sayer, Saer*

Scott (English) A man from Scotland *Scot, Scottie, Scotto, Scotty, Scotti, Scottey, Scottee, Scottea*

Sean (Irish) Form of John, meaning "God is gracious" *Shaughn, Shawn, Shaun, Shon, Shohn, Shonn, Shaundre, Shawnel*

Sebastian (Greek) The revered one *Sabastian, Seb, Sebastiano, Sebastien, Sebestyen, Sebo, Sebastyn, Sebestyen*

Sergio (Latin) An attendant; a servant *Seargeoh, Serge, Sergei, Sergeo, Sergey, Sergi, Sergios, Sergiu*

Seth (Hebrew) One who has been appointed *Sethe, Seath, Seathe, Zeth*

Shane (English) Form of John, meaning "God is gracious" *Shayn, Shayne, Shaine, Shain*

Shannon (Gaelic) Having ancient wisdom *Shanan, Shanen, Shannan, Shannen, Shanon*

Shea (Gaelic) An admirable man / from the fairy fortress *Shae, Shai, Shay, Shaye, Shaylon, Shays*

Sheffield (English) From the crooked field *Sheffeld*

Sheldon (English) From the steep valley *Shelden, Sheldan, Sheldun, Sheldin, Sheldyn, Shel*

Shepherd (English) One who herds sheep *Shepperd, Shep, Shepard, Shephard, Shepp, Sheppard*

Shields (Gaelic) A faithful protector *Sheelds, Shealds*

Shiloh (Hebrew) He who was sent *Shilo, Shyloh, Shylo*

Sierra (Spanish) From the jagged mountain range *Siera, Syerra, Syera, Seyera, Seeara*

Sigmund (German) The victorious protector *Siegmund, Sigmond, Zsigmond, Zygmunt*

Silas (Latin) Form of Silvanus, meaning "a woodland dweller"

Simon (Hebrew) God has heard *Shimon, Si, Sim, Samien, Semyon, Simen, Simeon, Simone*

Sinclair (English) Man from Saint Clair *Sinclaire, Sinclare, Synclair, Synclaire, Synclare*

Sirius (Greek) Resembling the brightest star *Syrius*

Smith (English) A blacksmith *Smyth, Smithe, Smythe, Smedt, Smid, Smitty, Smittee, Smittea*

Spencer (English) One who dispenses provisions *Spenser*

Stephen (Greek) Crowned with garland *Staffan, Steba, Steben, Stefan, Stefano, Steffan, Steffen, Steffon, Steven, Steve*

Sterling (English) One who is highly valued *Sterlyng, Stirling, Sterlyn*

Stuart (English) A steward; the keeper of the estate *Steward, Stewart, Stewert, Stuert, Stu, Stew*

Sully (English) From the southern meadow *Sulley, Sulli, Sullie, Sulleigh, Sullee, Sullea, Sulleah, Suthley*

Sullivan (Gaelic) Having dark eyes *Sullavan, Sullevan, Sullyvan*

Sylvester (Latin) Man from the forest *Silvester, Silvestre, Silvestro, Sylvestre, Sylvestro, Sly, Sevester, Seveste*

Sullivan

We chose my son's name purely because I really liked it. He's Sullivan, and not after any TV show, Irish heritage, or family names. It just came down to the fact that I thought Sully was really original. Letting my husband pick his middle name sealed the deal. —Ranae, MN

T

Taft (French / English) From the homestead / from the marshes *Tafte*

Taggart (Gaelic) Son of a priest *Taggert, Taggort, Taggirt, Taggyrt*

Tanner (English) One who makes leather *Tannere, Tannor, Tannar, Tannir, Tannyr, Tannur, Tannis*

Tate (English) A cheerful man; one who brings happiness to others *Tayt, Tayte, Tait, Taite, Taet, Taete*

Taylor (English) Cutter of cloth, one who alters garments

Teagan (Gaelic) A handsome man *Teegan, Teygan, Tegan, Teigan*

Ted (English) Form of Theodore, meaning "a gift from God" *Tedd, Teddy, Teddi, Teddie, Teddee, Teddea, Teddey, Tedric*

Terrance (Latin) From an ancient Roman clan *Tarrants, Tarrance, Tarrence, Tarrenz, Terencio, Terance, Terrence, Terrey, Terry*

Thackary (English) Form of Zachary, meaning "the Lord remembers" *Thackery, Thakary, Thakery, Thackari, Thackarie, Thackarey, Thackaree, Thackarea*

Thaddeus (Aramaic) Having heart *Tad, Tadd, Taddeo, Taddeusz, Thad, Thadd, Thaddaios, Thaddaos*

Thatcher (English) One who fixes roofs *Thacher, Thatch, Thatche, Thaxter, Thacker, Thaker, Thackere, Thakere*

Thayer (Teutonic) Of the nation's army

Theodore (Greek) A gift from God *Ted, Teddy, Teddie, Theo, Theodor*

Thomas (Aramaic) One of twins *Tam, Tamas, Tamhas, Thom, Thomason, Thomson, Thompson, Tomas*

Tiernan (Gaelic) Lord of the manor *Tiarnan, Tiarney, Tierney, Tierny, Tiernee, Tiernea, Tierni, Tiernie*

Timothy (Greek) One who honors God *Tim, Timmo, Timmothy, Timmy, Timo, Timofei, Timofeo*

Tobias (Hebrew) The Lord is good *Toby*

Todd (English) Resembling a fox *Tod*

Torrence (Gaelic) From the little hills *Torence, Torrance, Torrens, Torrans, Toran, Torran, Torrin, Torn, Torry*

Tracy (Gaelic) One who is warlike *Tracey, Traci, Tracie, Tracee, Tracea, Treacy, Trace, Tracen*

Travis (French) To cross over
Travys, Traver, Travers, Traviss,
Trevis, Trevys, Travus, Traves

Trenton (English) From the
town near the rushing rapids
Trent, Trynt, Trenten, Trentyn

Trevor (Welsh) From the large
village *Trefor, Trevar, Trever,*
Treabhar, Treveur, Trevir, Trevur

Trey (English) The third-born
child *Tre, Trai, Trae, Tray, Traye,*
Trayton, Treyton, Trayson

Tripp (English) A traveler
Trip, Trypp, Tryp, Tripper, Trypper

Tristan (Celtic) A sorrowful
man; in Arthurian legend, a
knight of the Round Table
Trystan, Tris, Tristam, Tristen,
Tristian, Tristin, Triston, Tristram

Troy (Gaelic) Son of a foot
soldier *Troye, Troi*

Tucker (English) One who
makes garments *Tuker,*
Tuckerman, Tukerman, Tuck,
Tuckman, Tukman, Tuckere,
Toukere

Tyler (English) A tiler of roofs
Tilar, Tylar, Tylor, Tiler, Tilor, Ty,
Tye, Tylere

Tyson (French) One who is
high-spirited; fiery *Thyssen,*
Tiesen, Tyce, Tycen, Tyeson,
Tyssen, Tysen, Tysan

U

Uberto (Italian) Form of Hubert, meaning "having a shining intellect" *Ulberto, Umberto*

Ulmer (German) Having the fame of the wolf *Ullmer, Ullmar, Ulmarr, Ullmarr, Ulfmer, Ulfmar, Ulfmaer*

Uri (Hebrew) Form of Uriah, meaning "the Lord is my light" *Urie, Ury, Urey, Uree, Urea*

Uriah (Hebrew) The Lord is my light *Uri, Uria, Urias, Urija, Urijah, Uriyah, Urjasz, Uriya*

Usher (Latin) From the mouth of the river *Ushar, Ushir, Ussher, Usshar, Usshir*

Uzi (Hebrew) Having great power *Uzie, Uzy, Uzey, Uzee, Uzea, Uzzi, Uzzie, Uzzy*

V

Valentine (Latin) One who is strong and healthy *Val, Valentin, Valentino, Valentyne, Ualan*

Vance (English) From the marshland *Vanse*

Vernon (French) From the alder-tree grove *Vern, Vernal, Vernard, Verne, Vernee, Vernen, Verney, Vernin*

Victor (Latin) One who is victorious; the champion *Vic, Vick, Victoriano*

Vidal (Spanish) A giver of life *Videl, Videlio, Videlo, Vidalo, Vidalio, Vidas*

Vincent (Latin) One who prevails; the conqueror *Vicente, Vicenzio, Vicenzo, Vin, Vince, Vincens, Vincente, Vincentius*

Virgil (Latin) The staff-bearer *Verge, Vergil, Vergilio, Virgilio, Vergilo, Virgilo, Virgilijus*

Vladimir (Slavic) A famous prince *Vladamir, Vladimeer, Vladimyr, Vladimyre, Vladamyr, Vladamyre, Vladameer, Vladimer*

W

> ···················· **Wade** ····················
>
> When I was preparing to leave the hospital with our new son, Wade, I told the nurses, "I'm ready to get Wade." The nurse pointed down the hall to the scale (weighed). I questioned our choice of the name for a moment, but now Wade enjoys writing his name instead of "weighed" on spelling tests. Teachers don't count it wrong after hearing his story!
> —Kay, NE

Wade (English) To cross the river ford *Wayde, Waid, Waide, Waddell, Wadell, Waydell, Waidell, Waed*

Walker (English) One who trods the cloth *Walkar, Walkir, Walkor*

Wainwright (English) One who builds wagons *Wainright, Wainewright, Wayneright, Waynewright, Waynwright*

Wallace (Scottish) A Welshman, a man from the South *Wallach, Wallas, Wallie, Wallis, Wally, Wlash, Welch*

Walter (German) The commander of the army *Walther, Walt, Walte, Walder, Wat, Wouter, Wolter, Woulter*

Warner (German) Of the defending army *Werner, Wernher, Warnher, Worner, Wornher*

Warren (English / German) From the fortress

Watson (English) The son of Walter *Watsin, Watsen, Watsan, Watkins, Watckins, Watkin, Watckin, Wattekinson*

Wayne (English) One who builds wagons *Wain, Wanye, Wayn, Waynell, Waynne, Guwayne*

Webster (English) A weaver *Weeb, Web, Webb, Webber, Weber, Webbestre, Webestre, Webbe*

Wendell (German) One who travels; a wanderer *Wendel, Wendale, Wendall, Wendele, Wendal, Windell, Windel, Windal*

Wesley (English) From the western meadow *Wes, Wesly, Wessley, Westleigh, Westley, Wesli, Weslie, Wesleigh*

Weston (English) From the western town

Wiley (English) One who is crafty; from the meadow by the water *Wily, Wileigh, Wili, Wilie, Wilee, Wylie, Wyly, Wyley*

William (German) The determined protector *Wilek, Wileck, Wilhelm, Wilhelmus, Wilkes, Wilkie, Wilkinson, Will, Guillaume, Quilliam*

Winston (English) Of the joy stone; from the friendly town *Win, Winn, Winsten, Winstonn, Wynstan, Wynsten, Wynston, Winstan*

Wyatt (English) Having the strength of a warrior *Wyat, Wyatte, Wyate, Wiatt, Wiatte, Wiat, Wiate, Wyeth*

William

William is a family name on my husband's side. My husband was the only boy in his family, and Will was supposed to be his son's name, and not one of his sisters' children. I agreed on one condition: that we would call him Will. Hopefully, he won't change it after I fought so hard to avoid Bill and Billy!
—Michelle, MO

X

Xakery (American) Form of Zachery, meaning "the Lord remembers" *Xaccary, Xaccery, Xach, Xacharie, Xachery, Xack, Xackarey, Xackary*

Xalvador (Spanish) Form of Salvador, meaning "a savior" *Xalvadore, Xalvadoro, Xalvadorio, Xalbador, Xalbadore, Xalbadorio, Xalbadoro, Xabat*

Xavier (Basque / Arabic) Owner of a new house / one who is bright *Xaver, Xever, Xabier, Xaviere, Xabiere, Xaviar, Xaviare, Xavior*

Xesus (Galician) Form of Jesus, meaning "God is my salvation"

Xoan (Galician) Form of John, meaning "God is gracious" *Xoane, Xohn, Xon*

Y

Yael (Israeli) Strength of God
Yaele

Yahweh (Hebrew) Refers
to God *Yahveh, Yaweh, Yaveh,
Yehowah, Yehweh, Yehoveh*

Yale (Welsh) From the fertile
upland *Yayle, Yayl, Yail, Yaile*

Yohan (German) Form of
John, meaning "God is
gracious" *Yohanan, Yohann,
Yohannes, Yohon, Yohonn,
Yohonan*

York (English) From the yew
settlement *Yorck, Yorc, Yorke*

Yves (French) A young archer
Yve, Yvo, Yvon, Yvan, Yvet, Yvete

Z

Zachariah (Hebrew) The Lord remembers *Zacaria, Zacarias, Zaccaria, Zaccariah, Zachaios, Zacharia, Zacharias, Zacherish*

Zachary (Hebrew) Form of Zachariah, meaning "the Lord remembers" *Zaccary, Zaccery, Zach, Zacharie, Zachery, Zack, Zackarey, Zackary, Thackary, Xakery*

Zander (Slavic) Form of Alexander, meaning "a helper and defender of mankind" *Zandros, Zandro, Zandar, Zandur, Zandre*

Zane (English) Form of John, meaning "God is gracious" *Zayne, Zayn, Zain, Zaine*

Zayden (Arabic) Form of Zayd, meaning "to become greater, to grow" *Zaiden*

Zeke (English) Form of Ezekiel, meaning "strengthened by God" *Zekiel, Zeek, Zeeke, Zeeq*

Zion (Hebrew) From the citadel *Zionn, Zione, Zionne*

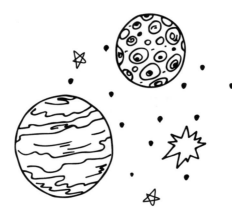

The Top 1,000

N eed some more options? Here are the recent top 1,000 boys names in the United States according to the Social Security Administration:

Aaden	Adrian	Alec	Allen
Aarav	Adriel	Alejandro	Alonso
Aaron	Adrien	Alessandro	Alonzo
Abdiel	Agustin	Alex	Alvaro
Abdullah	Ahmad	Alexander	Alvin
Abel	Ahmed	Alexis	Amari
Abraham	Aidan	Alexzander	Ameer
Abram	Aiden	Alfonso	Amir
Ace	Alan	Alfred	Amos
Achilles	Alaric	Alfredo	Anakin
Adam	Albert	Ali	Anders
Adan	Alberto	Alijah	Anderson
Aden	Alden	Alistair	Andre
Adonis	Aldo	Allan	Andres

Andrew	Atlas	Bentlee	Brayden
Andy	Atticus	Bentley	Braydon
Angel	August	Benton	Braylen
Angelo	Augustine	Billy	Braylon
Anson	Augustus	Bishop	Brayson
Anthony	Austin	Bjorn	Brecken
Anton	Avery	Blaine	Brendan
Antonio	Avi	Blaise	Brenden
Apollo	Axel	Blake	Brennan
Archer	Axl	Blaze	Brentley
Ares	Axton	Bo	Brett
Ari	Ayaan	Bobby	Brian
Arian	Ayan	Bodhi	Briar
Ariel	Ayden	Bodie	Bridger
Arjun	Aydin	Boone	Briggs
Arlo	Azariah	Boston	Brixton
Armando	Barrett	Bowen	Brock
Armani	Baylor	Braden	Brodie
Aron	Beau	Bradley	Brody
Arthur	Beckett	Brady	Bronson
Arturo	Beckham	Brandon	Brooks
Aryan	Ben	Branson	Bruce
Asa	Benjamin	Brantley	Bruno
Asher	Bennett	Braxton	Bryan
Ashton	Benson	Brayan	Bryant

Bryce	Carson	Clark	Crew
Brycen	Carter	Clay	Cristian
Brysen	Case	Clayton	Cristiano
Bryson	Casen	Clyde	Crosby
Byron	Casey	Cody	Cruz
Cade	Cash	Coen	Cullen
Caden	Cason	Cohen	Curtis
Caiden	Caspian	Colby	Cyrus
Cain	Cassius	Cole	Dakota
Cairo	Castiel	Coleman	Dallas
Caleb	Cayden	Colin	Dalton
Callan	Cayson	Collin	Damari
Callen	Cedric	Colson	Damian
Callum	Cesar	Colt	Damien
Calvin	Chad	Colten	Damon
Camden	Chaim	Colton	Dane
Camdyn	Chance	Conner	Dangelo
Cameron	Chandler	Connor	Daniel
Camilo	Channing	Conor	Danny
Camron	Charles	Conrad	Dante
Canaan	Charlie	Cooper	Darian
Cannon	Chase	Corbin	Dariel
Carl	Chris	Corey	Dario
Carlos	Christian	Cory	Darius
Carmelo	Christopher	Craig	Darrell

Darren	Diego	Edison	Enrique
Darwin	Dilan	Eduardo	Enzo
Dash	Dillon	Edward	Ephraim
Davian	Dimitri	Edwin	Eric
David	Dominic	Eli	Erick
Davion	Dominick	Elian	Erik
Davis	Dominik	Elias	Ernest
Dawson	Dominique	Eliezer	Ernesto
Dax	Donald	Elijah	Esteban
Daxton	Donovan	Eliseo	Ethan
Dayton	Dorian	Elisha	Eugene
Deacon	Douglas	Elliot	Evan
Dean	Drake	Elliott	Everett
Deandre	Draven	Ellis	Ezekiel
Decker	Drew	Emanuel	Ezequiel
Declan	Duke	Emerson	Ezra
Demetrius	Duncan	Emery	Fabian
Dennis	Dustin	Emiliano	Felipe
Denver	Dwayne	Emilio	Felix
Derek	Dylan	Emmanuel	Fernando
Derrick	Eason	Emmet	Finley
Desmond	Easton	Emmett	Finn
Devin	Eddie	Emmitt	Finnegan
Devon	Eden	Emory	Finnley
Dexter	Edgar	Enoch	Fisher

Fletcher	Gianluca	Harper	Ira
Flynn	Gianni	Harrison	Isaac
Ford	Gibson	Harry	Isaiah
Forrest	Gideon	Harvey	Isaias
Foster	Giovanni	Hassan	Ishaan
Fox	Gordon	Hayden	Ismael
Francis	Grady	Hayes	Israel
Francisco	Graham	Heath	Issac
Franco	Grant	Hector	Ivan
Frank	Graysen	Hendrix	Izaiah
Frankie	Grayson	Henrik	Jabari
Franklin	Gregory	Henry	Jace
Frederick	Grey	Hezekiah	Jack
Gabriel	Greysen	Holden	Jackson
Gael	Greyson	Houston	Jacob
Gage	Griffin	Howard	Jacoby
Gannon	Guillermo	Hudson	Jad
Garrett	Gunnar	Hugh	Jaden
Gary	Gunner	Hugo	Jadiel
Gatlin	Gustavo	Hunter	Jagger
Gavin	Hamza	Huxley	Jaiden
George	Hank	Ian	Jaime
Gerald	Harlan	Ibrahim	Jairo
Gerardo	Harley	Ignacio	Jake
Giancarlo	Harold	Iker	Jakob

Jalen	Jayceon	Johan	Julio
Jamal	Jayden	John	Julius
Jamari	Jaylen	Johnathan	Junior
James	Jayson	Johnny	Justice
Jameson	Jaziel	Jon	Justin
Jamie	Jedidiah	Jonah	Kace
Jamir	Jefferson	Jonas	Kade
Jamison	Jeffery	Jonathan	Kaden
Jared	Jeffrey	Jordan	Kai
Jase	Jensen	Jordy	Kaiden
Jasiah	Jeremiah	Jorge	Kairo
Jason	Jeremias	Jose	Kaiser
Jasper	Jeremy	Joseph	Kaison
Javier	Jermaine	Joshua	Kaleb
Javion	Jerome	Josiah	Kalel
Javon	Jerry	Josue	Kamari
Jax	Jesse	Jovanni	Kamden
Jaxen	Jessie	Joziah	Kameron
Jaxon	Jesus	Juan	Kamryn
Jaxson	Jett	Judah	Kane
Jaxton	Jimmy	Jude	Kannon
Jaxx	Joaquin	Judson	Kareem
Jaxxon	Joe	Juelz	Karson
Jay	Joel	Julian	Karter
Jayce	Joey	Julien	Kase

Kasen	Kieran	Kyrie	Leo
Kash	Killian	Kyson	Leon
Kashton	King	Lachlan	Leonard
Kason	Kingsley	Lamar	Leonardo
Kayden	Kingston	Lance	Leonel
Kaysen	Knox	Landen	Leonidas
Kayson	Koa	Landon	Leroy
Keagan	Kobe	Landry	Levi
Keanu	Koda	Landyn	Lewis
Keaton	Kody	Lane	Liam
Keegan	Kohen	Langston	Lincoln
Keenan	Kole	Larry	Lionel
Keith	Kolten	Lawrence	Lochlan
Kellan	Kolton	Lawson	Logan
Kellen	Konnor	Layne	London
Kelvin	Korbin	Layton	Lorenzo
Kendall	Kristian	Leandro	Louie
Kendrick	Kristopher	Ledger	Louis
Kenneth	Kye	Lee	Luca
Kenny	Kylan	Legend	Lucas
Kevin	Kyle	Leif	Lucca
Khalid	Kylen	Leighton	Lucian
Khalil	Kyler	Leland	Luciano
Khari	Kyng	Lennon	Luis
Kian	Kyree	Lennox	Luka

Lukas	Markus	Mayson	Musa
Luke	Marley	Mekhi	Mustafa
Lyle	Marlon	Melvin	Myles
Lyric	Marshall	Memphis	Nash
Mack	Martin	Merrick	Nasir
Madden	Marvin	Messiah	Nathan
Maddox	Mason	Micah	Nathanael
Maddux	Mateo	Michael	Nathaniel
Magnus	Mathew	Micheal	Nehemiah
Maison	Mathias	Miguel	Neil
Major	Matias	Mike	Nelson
Makai	Matteo	Milan	Nicholas
Malachi	Matthew	Miles	Nickolas
Malakai	Matthias	Miller	Nico
Malcolm	Maurice	Milo	Nicolas
Malik	Mauricio	Misael	Niko
Manuel	Maverick	Mitchell	Nikolai
Marc	Max	Mohamed	Nikolas
Marcel	Maxim	Mohammad	Nixon
Marcelo	Maximilian	Mohammed	Noah
Marco	Maximiliano	Moises	Noe
Marcos	Maximo	Morgan	Noel
Marcus	Maximus	Moses	Nolan
Mario	Maxton	Moshe	Nova
Mark	Maxwell	Muhammad	Oakley

Odin	Prince	Reid	Rohan
Oliver	Princeton	Reign	Roland
Omar	Quentin	Remington	Roman
Omari	Quincy	Remy	Romeo
Orion	Quinn	Rene	Ronald
Orlando	Quinton	Reuben	Ronan
Oscar	Rafael	Rex	Ronin
Otis	Raiden	Rey	Ronnie
Otto	Ramiro	Reyansh	Rory
Owen	Ramon	Rhett	Rowan
Pablo	Randall	Rhys	Rowen
Parker	Randy	Ricardo	Roy
Patrick	Raphael	Richard	Royal
Paul	Rashad	Ricky	Royce
Paxton	Raul	Ridge	Ruben
Payton	Ray	Riley	Rudy
Pedro	Rayan	River	Russell
Peter	Rayden	Robert	Ryan
Peyton	Raylan	Roberto	Ryder
Philip	Raymond	Rocco	Ryker
Phillip	Reagan	Rocky	Rylan
Phoenix	Reece	Rodney	Ryland
Pierce	Reed	Rodrigo	Sage
Porter	Reese	Rogelio	Salvador
Preston	Reginald	Roger	Salvatore

Sam	Simon	Terrence	Tristian
Samir	Sincere	Terry	Troy
Samson	Skylar	Thaddeus	Tucker
Samuel	Skyler	Thatcher	Ty
Santana	Solomon	Theo	Tyler
Santiago	Sonny	Theodore	Tyson
Santino	Soren	Thiago	Ulises
Santos	Spencer	Thomas	Uriah
Saul	Stanley	Timothy	Uriel
Sawyer	Stefan	Titan	Valentin
Scott	Stephen	Titus	Valentino
Seamus	Sterling	Tobias	Van
Sean	Stetson	Toby	Vance
Sebastian	Steven	Tomas	Vaughn
Sergio	Sullivan	Tommy	Vicente
Seth	Sutton	Tony	Victor
Shane	Sylas	Trace	Vihaan
Shaun	Tadeo	Travis	Vincent
Shawn	Talon	Trent	Vincenzo
Shepard	Tanner	Trenton	Vivaan
Shepherd	Tate	Trevor	Wade
Shiloh	Tatum	Trey	Walker
Shmuel	Taylor	Tripp	Walter
Silas	Terrance	Tristan	Warren
Simeon	Terrell	Tristen	Waylon

Wayne	Wilson	Yosef	Zander
Wells	Winston	Yousef	Zane
Wesley	Wyatt	Yusuf	Zavier
Wesson	Xander	Zachariah	Zayd
Westin	Xavier	Zachary	Zayden
Westley	Xzavier	Zackary	Zayn
Weston	Yadiel	Zahir	Zayne
Wilder	Yahir	Zaid	Zechariah
Will	Yahya	Zaiden	Zeke
William	Yehuda	Zain	Zion
Willie	Yisroel	Zaire	Zyaire

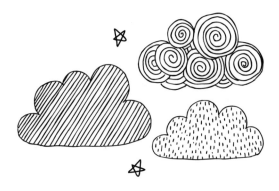

My Favorite Names ♡

....
....
....
....
....
....
....
....
....
....
....
....
....
....
....
....
....
....
....
....
....
....
....
....

My Favorite Names ♡

....
....
....
....
....
....
....
....
....
....
....
....
....
....
....
....
....
....
....
....
....
....
....

My Favorite Names ♡

....

....

....

....

....

....

....

....

....

....

....

....

....

....

....

....

....

....

....

....

....

....

Favorite Names ♡

My Favorite Names ♡

....

....

....

....

....

....

....

....

....

....

....

....

....

....

....

....

....

....

....

....

....

....

My Favorite Names ♡

....
....
....
....
....
....
....
....
....
....
....
....
....
....
....
....
....
....
....
....
....
....
....

My Favorite Names ♡

Favorite Names ♡

....

....

....

....

....

....

....

....

....

....

....

....

....

....

....

....

....

....

....

....

....

....

My Favorite Names ♡

....
....
....
....
....
....
....
....
....
....
....
....
....
....
....
....
....
....
....
....
....

My Favorite Names ♥

My Favorite Names ♡

....

....

....

....

....

....

....

....

....

....

....

....

....

....

....

....

....

....

....

....

....

....

....

My Favorite Names ♡

My Favorite Names ♡

....
....
....
....
....
....
....
....
....
....
....
....
....
....
....
....
....
....
....
....
....
....
....

My Favorite Names ♡

My Favorite Names ♡

....

....

....

....

....

....

....

....

....

....

....

....

....

....

....

....

....

....

....

....

....

....

....

My Favorite Names ♡